Bile Duct Cancer

Edited by Luis Rodrigo

Published in London, United Kingdom

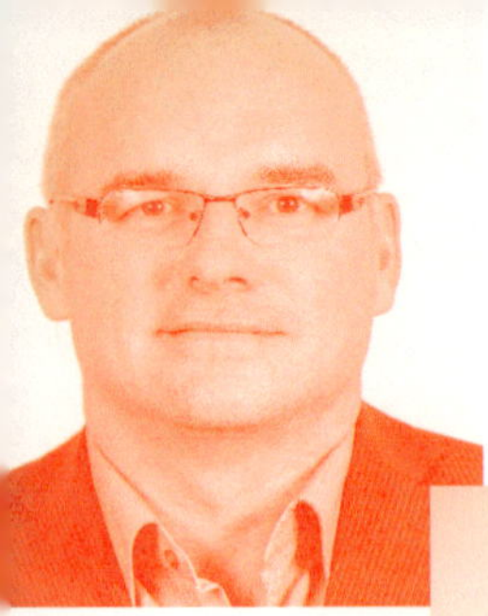
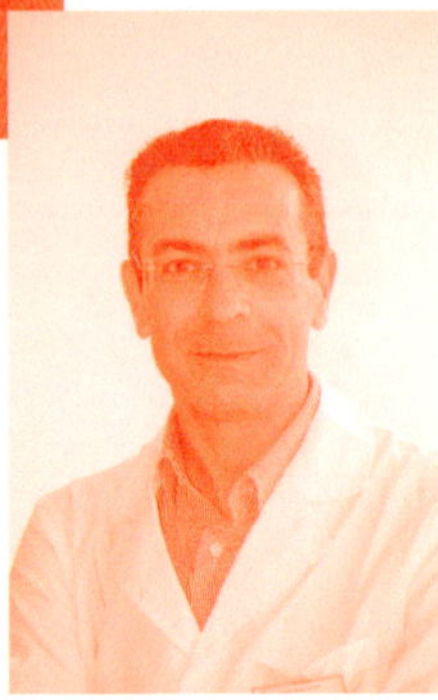
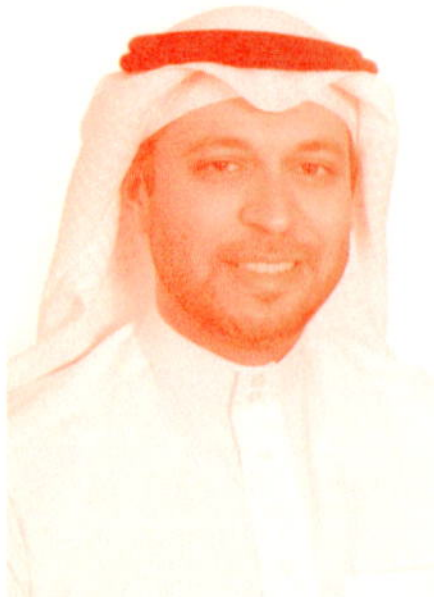
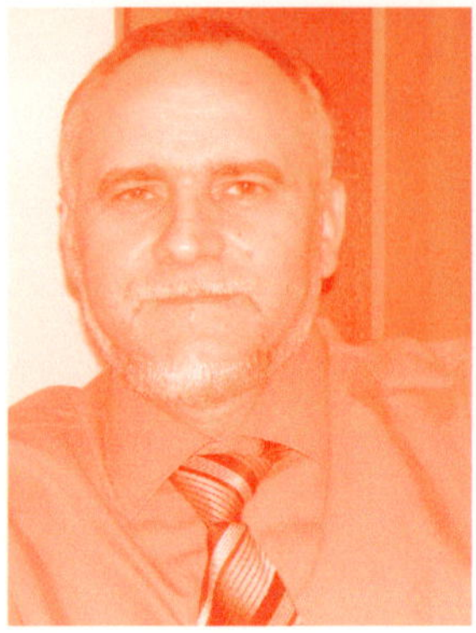
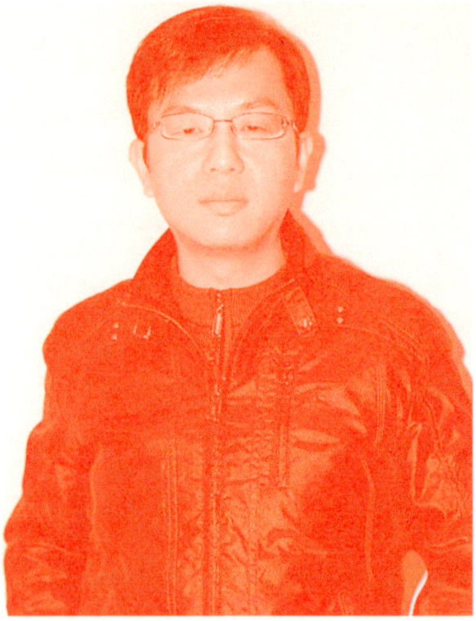
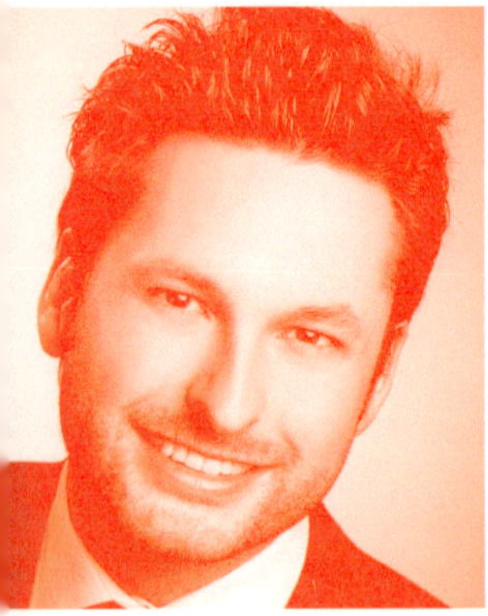
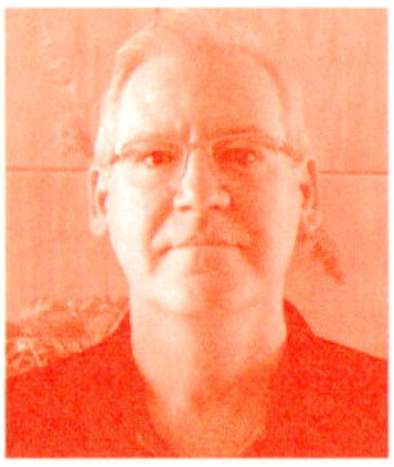

IntechOpen

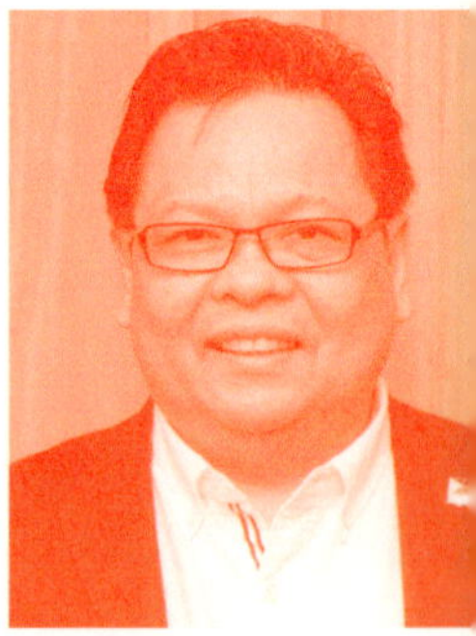
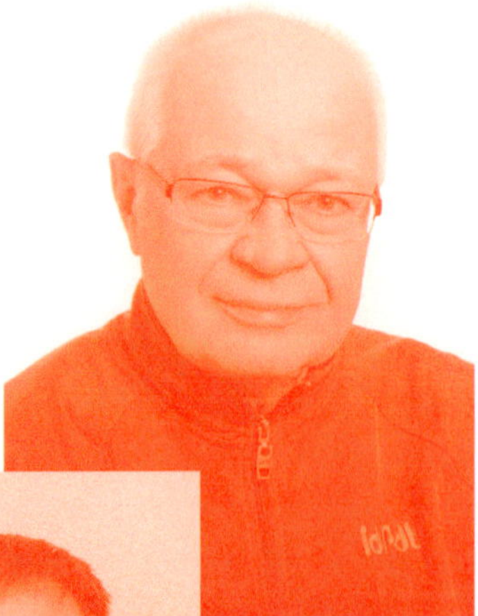
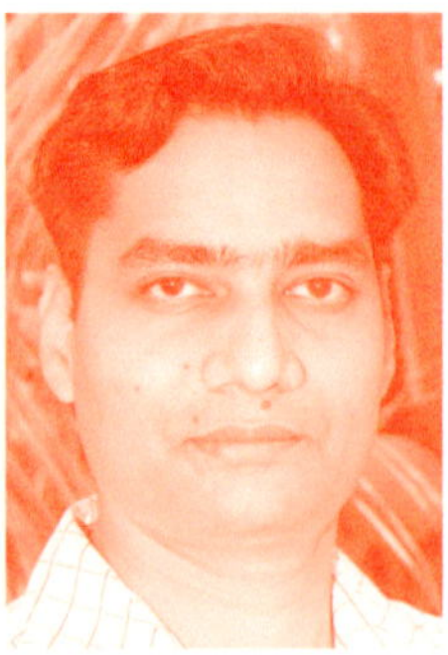
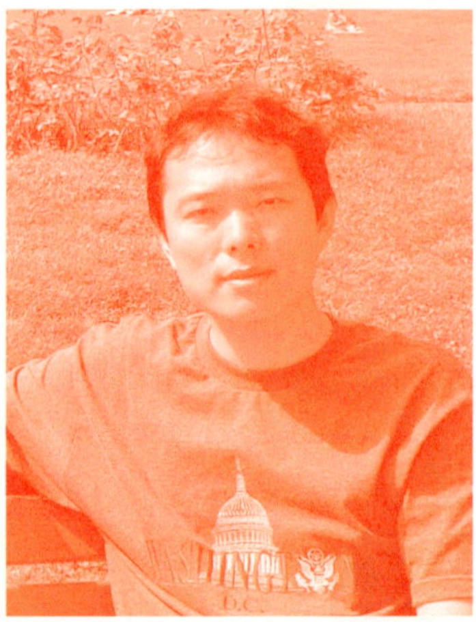
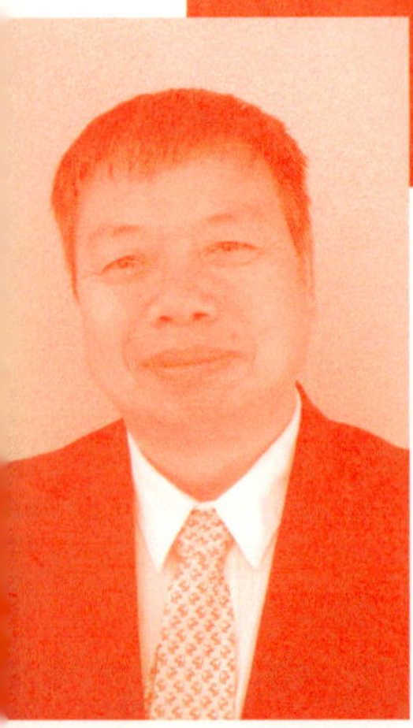
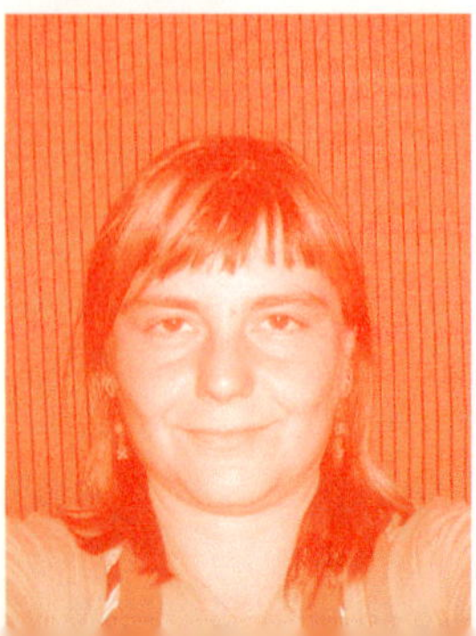

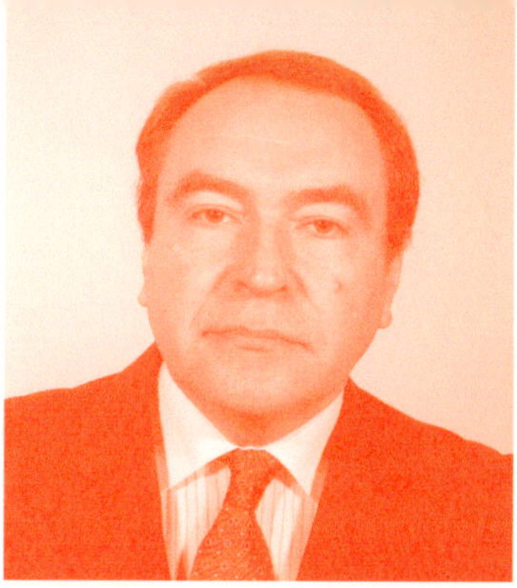
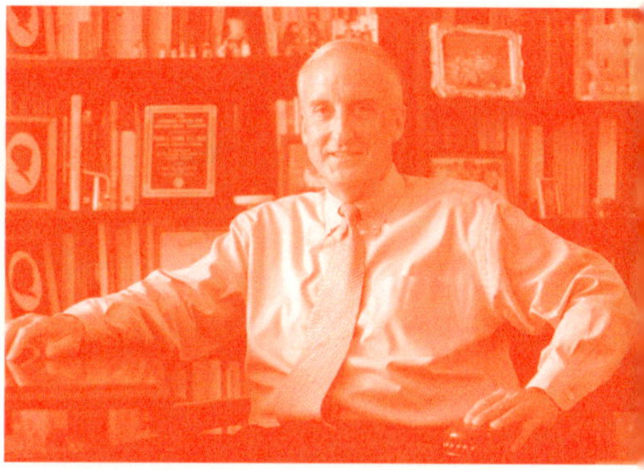
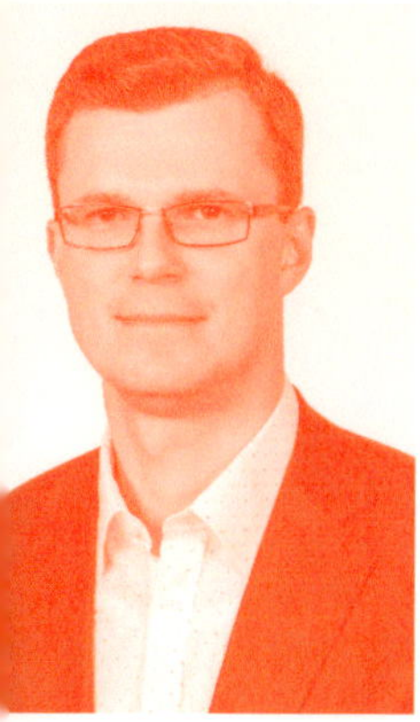
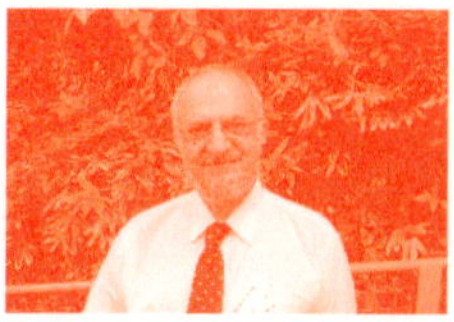
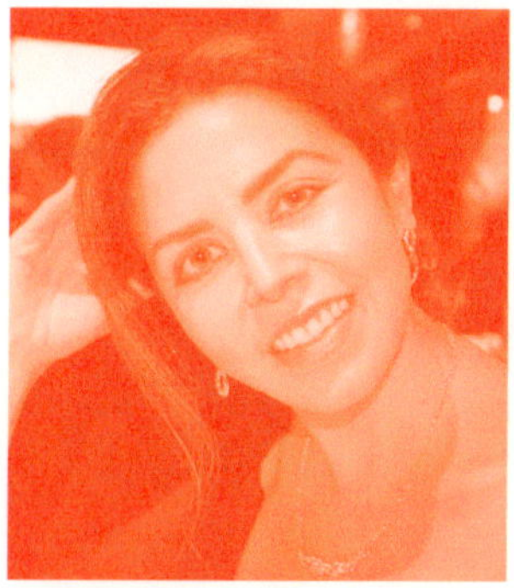

Supporting open minds since 2005

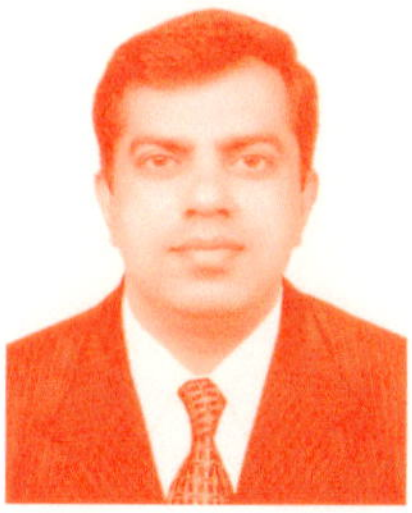
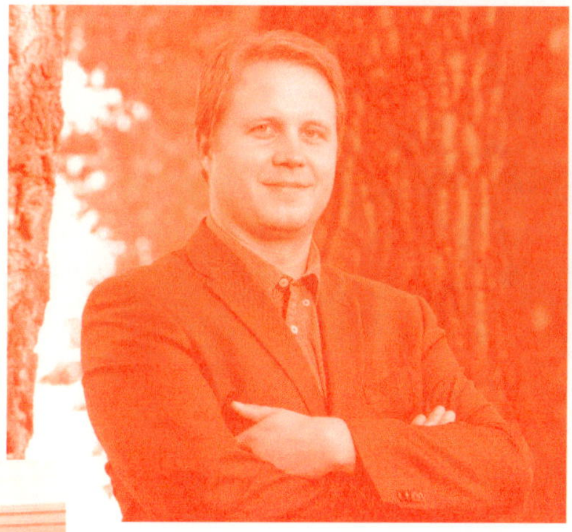
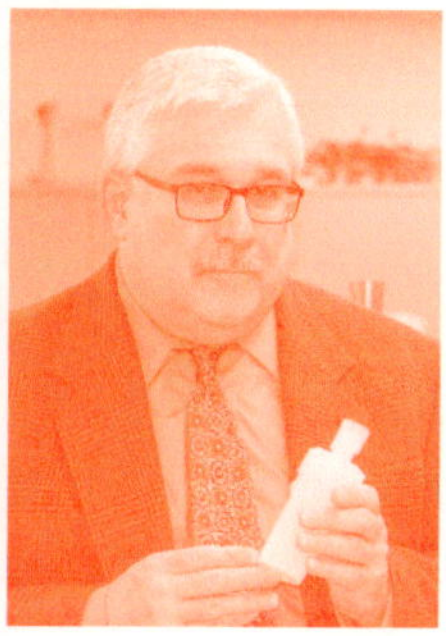
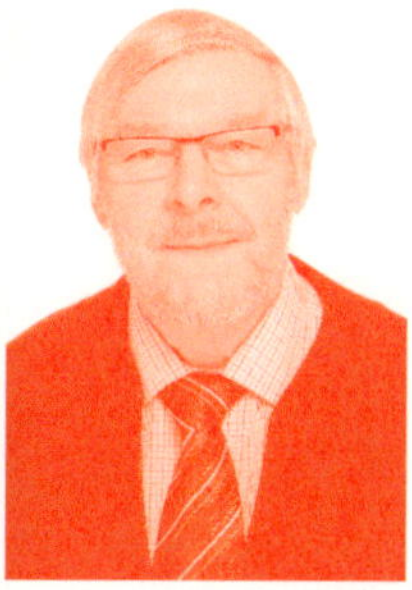
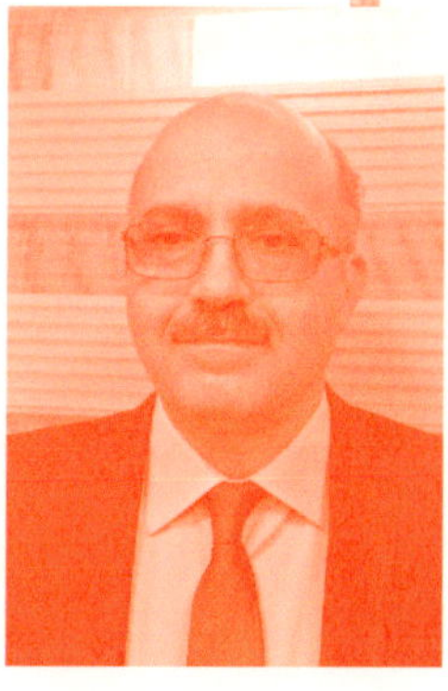
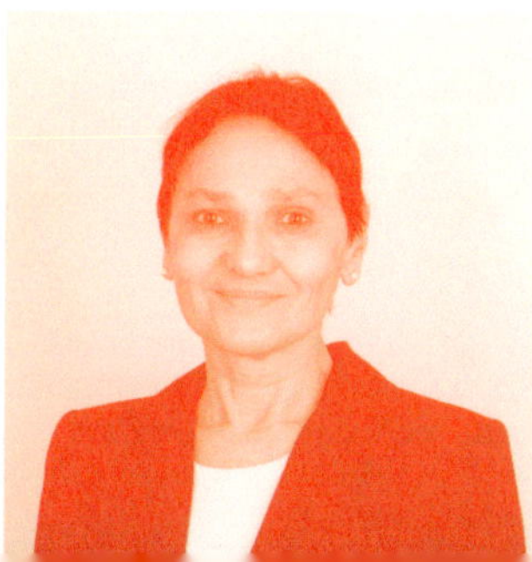
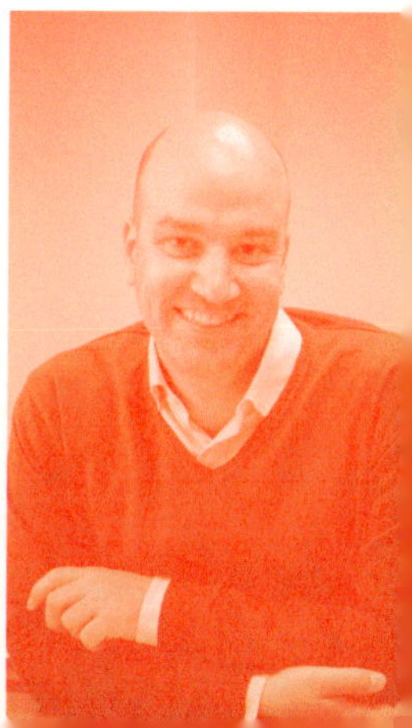

Bile Duct Cancer
http://dx.doi.org/10.5772/intechopen.78186
Edited by Luis Rodrigo

Contributors
Toshifumi Wakai, Pankaj Prasoon, Kohei Miura, Kizuki Yuza, Yuki Hirose, Jun Sakata, Ahmad A Madkhali, Faisal Al-Alem, Marco Massani, Tommaso Stecca, Bruno Pauletti, Ezio Caratozzolo, Luca Bonariol, Adrian Bartos, Andrei Herdean, Dana Monica Bartos, Gustavo Gomez, Fernando Hernandez, Nicolae Bacalbasa, Irina Balescu, Luis Rodrigo, Adolfo Suarez

First published in London, United Kingdom, 2019 by IntechOpen
IntechOpen is the global imprint of INTECHOPEN LIMITED, registered in England and Wales, registration number: 11086078, The Shard, 25th floor, 32 London Bridge Street
London, SE19SG - United Kingdom
Printed in Croatia

British Library Cataloguing-in-Publication Data
A catalogue record for this book is available from the British Library

Additional hard and PDF copies can be obtained from orders@intechopen.com

Bile Duct Cancer
Edited by Luis Rodrigo
p. cm.
Print ISBN 978-1-78923-875-4
Online ISBN 978-1-78923-876-1
eBook (PDF) ISBN 978-1-83962-215-1

For EU product safety concerns:
IN TECH d.o.o., Prolaz Marije Krucifikse Kozulić 3, 51000 Rijeka, Croatia, info@intechopen.com or visit our website at intechopen.com.

Meet the editor

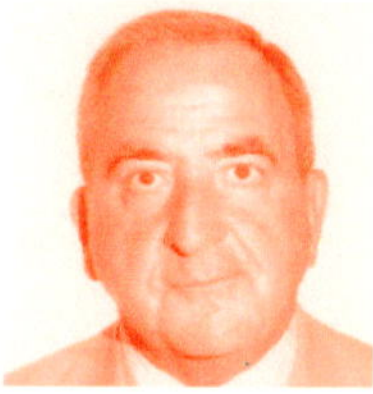

Dr. Luis Rodrigo MD is Emeritus Professor of Medicine at the University of Oviedo (Spain). He was Chief of Gastroenterology Service at the HUCA Hospital in Oviedo for more than 40 years. He obtained his PhD in 1975 and has developed a long teaching and research career. He has published a total of 585 scientific papers, 301 in English and the remainder in Spanish. He has participated as the main investigator in a total of 45 clinical trials and has directed 40 doctoral theses. He has contributed actively to the formation of around 100 specialisms in gastroenterology in hospitals both in Spain and abroad. He has written around 35 chapters in books on several subjects and is the editor of 22 books specializing in gastroenterology and related diseases.

Contents

Preface

It is a great honor and a pleasure for me to introduce *Bile Duct Cancer*, a new book about the variety of malignant tumors that occur throughout the biliary tree in the human body.

These tumors are typified by cholangiocarcinoma, their most common form. Its incidence is low compared with other malignancies, with only 1–2 cases per 100,000 inhabitants per year in developed countries, and it predominantly affects people older than 60 years. The tumor can occur in any part of the biliary tree, obstructing the flow of bile, giving rise to its most common clinical sign, the presence of persistent jaundice. In a small proportion of cases, there are some predisposing associated conditions, such as primary sclerosing cholangitis, choledochal cysts, and chronic infection by *Clonorchis sinensis* parasites. The main treatment is surgical resection. Patients generally have a poor prognosis.

The first section of the book includes an introductory chapter, by Dr. Luis Rodrigo and Dr. Adolfo Suarez, describing the general characteristics of these tumors.

Other sections are devoted to a range of aspects, such as the preoperative biliary techniques of drainage, a very controversial subject, including a wide range of endoscopic and percutaneous techniques, each with their advantages and drawbacks, beautifully described by Dr. Gustavo Gomez and Dr. Marco Massani in their separate chapters.

In another fascinating section, Dr. Nicolae Bacalbasa and his colleagues describe gallbladder carcinoma and the surgical aspects of its treatment.

The next section, by Dr. Wakai Toshifumi and his team, covers peri-hilar and hilar cholangiocarcinomas, which give rise to particular problems, not only from a diagnostic point of view, but also with respect to those regarding the surgical approach and the complete elimination of the tumor.

In the final section, Dr. Adrian Bartos and Dr. Ahmad Madkhali outline the characteristics of distal bile duct tumors, touching on aspects of the diagnosis and treatment of this type of cancer, which usually requires a duodenopancreatectomy to be carried out.

I would like to thank all the authors for their excellent contributions, and the IntechOpen editorial team, especially Ms. Anita Čondić and Ms. Dolores Kuzelj, for their cooperation and generous support throughout the preparation and editing of this book.

Luis Rodrigo, MD
Professor,
Emeritus Professor of Medicine,
University of Oviedo,
Oviedo, Spain

Section 1

Introduction

Chapter 1

Introductory Chapter: Bile Duct Cancer

Luis Rodrigo and Adolfo Suarez

1. Epidemiology and associated diseases

Cholangiocarcinoma (CC) is the most characteristic malignant tumour affecting to the bile ducts. It is a rare neoplasm that originates in the cells of the biliary epithelium. In the USA, it has a mean incidence of 1 case/100,000 inhabitants/year.

They are classified into three groups, with respect to their location within the biliary tree: (1) intrahepatic, (2) the upper and middle thirds and (3) the distal part of the common bile duct.

Intrahepatic tumours are the least frequent. They behave like primary hepatic tumours. Perihilar, or Klatskin, tumours are the most frequent, accounting for 60–80% of the total.

Their incidence increases with age, more cases appearing in patients aged between 50 and 70 years, with a clear predominance in men.

The diseases most frequently associated with it are primary sclerosing cholangitis (PSC), choledochal cysts, chronic infections with the parasite *Clonorchis sinensis* (typical of Asian countries and with a predominant intrahepatic location) and the presence of cholelithiasis and choledocholithiasis. The presence of PSC is an important risk factor, given that it occurs in 30% of cases. In many patients, no known risk factors are found.

2. Clinical presentation

Presentation depends fundamentally on the location of the tumour, although more than 90% of cases exhibit obstructive jaundice as their main sign. Other associated symptoms are episodes of cholangitis (which occur frequently after manipulation of the biliary tract), weight loss, abdominal pain, rebel pruritus and altered liver function test values, with elevated serum levels of bilirubin, alkaline phosphatase (AP) and gamma-glutamyl transpeptidase (GGT).

Transaminases can be quite elevated. The levels of serum tumour markers type CEA and CA 19-9 are usually raised, although they are of little diagnostic use due to their lack of sensitivity and specificity for this purpose. There are currently no other markers available that are useful for diagnosing or following up these tumours.

3. Diagnostic procedures

Abdominal ultrasound (AU) produces results of varying quality, depending on the location of the tumour. Distal tumours can be confused with primary pancreatic or periampullary neoplasms. Hilar tumours are usually infiltrative, characteristically causing dilation of the intrahepatic bile duct and collapse of the extrahepatic duct.

Computerised axial tomography (CAT) can help identify the type and stage of an existing tumour.

Magnetic resonance cholangiography (MRC) is the current imaging technique of choice for studying the bile duct, providing information simultaneously about the bile duct and its locoregional extension.

Endoscopic ultrasound (EU) is especially useful in tumours located in the distal third of the duct, enabling the tumour to be sampled and its cytology determined.

Endoscopic retrograde cholangiopancreatography (ERCP) and percutaneous cholangiography (PC) are currently reserved for the palliative treatment of obstructive jaundice, through the placement of biliary prostheses.

4. Classification

The classification of bile duct tumours is controversial and complex. Perihilar tumours are customarily divided into four types, depending on their extension and type of surgical resection, following the Bismuth-Corlette classification [1–3].

The working group of the Memorial Sloan-Kettering Cancer Center in New York has proposed a new classification that is better correlated with the prognosis, but which is very complex and does not take into account the current concepts of resectability.

In general, it is considered appropriate to separate perihilar tumours and those of the distal bile duct into separate groups.

5. Treatment

Resectability is determined by the absence of metastases, including retropancreatic nodes, non-invasion of the great vessels and the possibility of performing a surgical resection with free margins. Some groups recommend to do an exploratory laparoscopy prior to the indication of surgery, to rule out the presence of dissemination.

The discovery of lymph node involvement below the hepatoduodenal ligament indicates inoperability.

The placement of a biliary prosthesis before surgery is controversial. While some groups consider that it ameliorates the jaundice, allows the collection of biopsies and facilitates access to the bile duct after surgery, others postulate that it makes complications, especially cholangitis, more likely to arise [4–6].

The type of resection depends on the location of the tumour. In distal tumours, a cephalic duodenopancreatectomy is performed. This should be carried out in a reference centre to reduce the likelihood of perioperative morbidity (30%).

In hilar lesions, the resection should be individualised with respect to the extent of the tumour. A liver resection should normally be carried out that includes segments IV and V, extended according to the size of the tumour mass in order to ensure disease-free resection margins.

Liver transplantation is not a feasible therapeutic option because of the high rate of recurrence that occurs during follow-up.

In cases in which resection is not possible, it is advisable to drain the bile duct through catheters that are carefully placed through endoscopy or inserted percutaneously. Endoscopic drainage is considered easier and safer in distal tumours, while the percutaneous approach is more effective in proximal tumours. The most common short-term complication is cholangitis, although this can be prevented by giving antibiotics before placement. In the long term, the obstruction of the prosthesis, either by tumour progression, biliary detritus or food debris, prevents the flow of bile through the duct, and the jaundice reappears.

There is currently not enough scientific evidence available to make firm recommendations about the use of adjuvant therapy after surgery. The Guidelines of the European Society of Medical Oncology (ESMO) suggest the use of chemotherapy and/or palliative radiotherapy after non-curative resections and of chemoradiotherapy after curative resections.

Neoadjuvant therapy is not usually recommended because of the deterioration that patients usually present at the time of diagnosis [7–10].

6. Prognosis and prevention

The prognosis of bile duct cancer is bad. Malignant tumours of the bile duct are usually diagnosed at advanced stages, with infiltration of neighbouring organs such as the liver, gallbladder, adjoining vessels and distant metastases, which often contraindicates surgery. Average survival is 12–24 months. Distal tumours have a better prognosis, with a 5-year survival of 15–25%.

Screening programmes have not proved to be effective for the early detection of these tumours. However, in carriers of PSC, it is advisable to undertake periodic surveillance using imaging techniques (e.g. MRC) and the determination of CA 19-9 serum levels, although none of these procedures is sufficiently specific [11, 12].

Author details

Luis Rodrigo* and Adolfo Suarez
Hospital Universitario Central de Asturias (HUCA), Oviedo, Spain

*Address all correspondence to: lrodrigosaez@gmail.com

References

[1] Paul A, Kaiser GM, Molmenti EP, Scroeder T, Vernadakis S, Oezcelik A, et al. Klatskin tumors and the accuracy of the Bismuth-Corlette classification. The American Surgeon. 2011;**77**:1695-1699

[2] Li B, Xiong XZ, Zhou Y, Wu SJ, You Z, Lu J, et al. Prognostic value of lymphovascular invasion in Bismuth-Corlette type IV hilar cholangiocarcinoma. World Journal of Gastroenterology. 2017;**23**:6685-6693

[3] Ji GW, Zhu FP, Wang K, Jiao CY, Shao ZC, Li XC. Clinical implications of biliary confluence pattern for Bismuth-Corlette type IV hilar cholangiocarcinoma applied to hemi-hepatectomy. Journal of Gastrointestinal Surgery. 2017;**21**:666-675

[4] Coelen RJS, Roos E, Wiggers JK, Besselink MG, Buis CL, Busch ORC, et al. Endoscopic versus percutaneous biliary drainage in patients with resectable perihilar cholangiocarcinoma: A multicenter randomised controlled trial. The Lancet Gastroenterology & Hepatology. 2018;**3**:681-690

[5] Tang Z, Yang Y, Meng W, Li X. Best option for preoperative drainage in Klatskin tumor: A systematic review and meta-analysis. Medicine (Baltimore). 2017;**96**:e8372

[6] Hameed A, Pang T, Chiou J, Pleass H, Lam V, Hollands M, et al. Percutaneous vs. endoscopic pre-operative biliary drainage in hilar cholangiocarcinoma. A systematic review and meta-analysis. HPB: The Official Journal of the International Hepato Pancreato Biliary Association. 2016;**18**:400-410

[7] Esnaola NF, Meyer JE, Karachristos A, Maranki JL, Camp ER, Denlinger CS. Evaluation and management of intrahepatic and extrahepatic cholangiocarcinoma. Cancer. 2016;**122**:1349-1369

[8] Nakano M, Ariizumi SI, Yamamoto M. Intrahepatic cholangiocarcinoma. Seminars in Diagnostic Pathology. 2017;**34**:160-166

[9] Waseem D, Tushar P. Intrahepatic, perihilar and distal cholangiocarcinoma: Management and outcomes. Annals of Hepatology. 2017;**16**:133-139

[10] Chun YS, Javie M. Systemic and adjuvant therapies for intrahepatic cholangiocarcinoma. Cancer Control. 2017;**24**:1073274817729241

[11] Kim HJ, Kim JS, Joo MK, Lee BJ, Yeon JE, Park JJ, et al. Hepatolithiasis and intrahepatic cholangiocarcinoma: A review. World Journal of Gastroenterology. 2015;**21**:13418-13431

[12] Buisson Y. Control of *Opisthorchis viverrini* infection for cholangiocarcinoma prevention. Bulletin de la Société de Pathologie Exotique. 2017;**110**:61-67

Section 2

Preoperative Biliary Drainage

Chapter 2

Preoperative Biliary Drainage: Methods, Advantages, and Complications

Gómez-Torres Gustavo Ángel
and Hernández-García Fernando Santiago

Abstract

Malignant biliary obstruction is very difficult to treat; only 10–20% of the patients are suitable for curative resections. Obstructive jaundice is associated with a pro-inflammatory state, altering the normal physiology and affecting multiple organ systems. So, patients with malignant obstructive jaundice are at increased risk of postoperative complications. Nevertheless, the preoperative biliary drainage (PBD) remains controversial, because the procedures themselves can be associated with septic and other complications. The main therapeutic options for PBD in malignant biliary obstruction are percutaneous biliary drainage and endoscopic biliary drainage. The knowledge of the approaches, their advantages, and complications are essential for the management of patients with pathologies that produce biliary obstruction such as bile duct cancer. The aim of this chapter is to review the methods for biliary drainage and its indications, advantages, and complications.

Keywords: biliary drainage, obstructive jaundice, cholangiocarcinoma, endoscopic biliary drainage, percutaneous biliary drainage

1. Introduction

Malignant obstructive jaundice is a common condition caused by various adenocarcinomas, including cholangiocarcinoma [1–7]. Hilar cholangiocarcinoma, which is also known as Klatskin's tumor, accounts for about 50% of cholangiocarcinoma cases [3, 8]. Due to the silent tumor growth, curative resection is often not suitable at diagnosis. Only 10–20% of cases will be candidates for curative resection [1, 2].

Biliary obstruction from cholangiocarcinoma has been identified as an important risk factor for postoperative mortality. Biliary obstruction alters the normal physiology and affects multiple organ systems and can lead to jaundice, coagulopathy, and hepatic and renal dysfunction [2, 9–11]. Jaundice has been recognized as a major risk factor for performing pancreatic and liver surgery [12]. The presence of toxic substances such as bilirubin and bile salts, impaired liver function, and altered nutritional status has been proposed as responsible factors for increased infectious complications. Evidence suggests that biliary drainage may improve immune function and nutritional status and reduce the risk of infection [2, 13].

Despite these apparent advantages of performing a preoperative biliary drainage, the safety of the conventional preoperative biliary drainage has not been widely acknowledged, and the benefit remains controversial [3, 14]. Endoscopic biliary drainage (EBD) and percutaneous transhepatic biliary drainage (PTBD) are the two preoperative biliary drainage procedures available [2, 15]. Endoscopic drainage methods may be more suitable for type I and II tumors, while type III and IV tumors may be more easily drained percutaneously; nevertheless, there is not a guideline, and no consensus has been reached about the preferred approach, so the choice is usually made according to the local expertise and availability [5, 15]. Thus, the knowledge of the approaches, their advantages, and complications are essential for the management of patients with pathologies that produce biliary obstruction such as the bile duct cancer. The aim of this chapter is to review the methods for biliary drainage and its indications.

1.1 Indications

Obstruction of the bile duct: pancreatic neoplasm, cholangiocarcinoma, and gallbladder neoplasm.

The target of the biliary drainage is:

- Relieve obstructive jaundice
- Complications of biliary obstruction as cholangitis or sepsis
- Palliative treatment in patients not candidates for surgery
- Biopsy, stent placement, and brachytherapy

Currently, drainage of the bile duct is accepted in the preoperative period of icteric patients with poor general condition, bilirubin >10 mg/dl, and those patients who are going to undergo neoadjuvant treatment [5, 13].

2. Endoscopic biliary drainage

There are two techniques for endoscopic biliary drainage, internal with endoscopic retrograde cholangiopancreatography (ERCP) and with external drainage performing endoscopic nasobiliary drainage (ENBD). Endoscopic transpapillary biliary drainage was first introduced by Soehendra and Reynders-Frederix [16]. Initially, only plastic stents were available, with the largest available stent being 11.5 Fr. Nowadays, uncovered metal stents became available, and multiple trials showed that self-expanded uncovered metal stents were associated with lower stent failure and cholangitis [15, 16].

Transpapillary stent placement with endoscopic retrograde cholangiopancreatography has been the preferred treatment modality for the palliation of malignant distal biliary obstruction [3, 19]. However, the performance in patients with resectable tumors is unclear. Most of the patients referred to speciality centers for surgical treatment have already undergone endoscopic drainage before referral [20]. But, a wide array of complications stemming from the procedure as pancreatitis, cholangitis, and stent dysfunction in untimely reintervention has continued to present a significant challenge [9, 19].

2.1 Technique

Before the procedure, it is important to perform image studies such as computed tomography or magnetic resonance to assess biliary anatomy and plan the approach for intervention. It is important to evaluate the risk of cholangitis in each patient, and we suggest administrating broad-spectrum antibiotics prior to the procedure. Using a therapeutic duodenoscope, the bile duct is selectively cannulated using a wire-guided sphincterotome. After a retrograde cholangiography is performed to localize the site of obstruction, the guide wire is maneuvered through and above the biliary stenosis followed by a catheter. The endoprosthesis is then pushed in position over the catheter (**Figure 1**) [17, 18].

2.1.1 ENBD

A guide wire is passed down the endoscope channel and through the bile duct, and the tip is advanced and looped high in the common hepatic duct or liver. A suitable drainage tube is then advanced through the endoscope to the tip of the wire. The guide wire is withdrawn, and the proximal end of the tube is rerouted from the mouth to the nose using temporary nasopharyngeal intubation.

2.2 Advantages

In addition to achieving imaging of the biliary duct and biliary drainage, endoscopic biliary drainage is also used for tissue diagnosis using brush cytology or fine-needle aspiration, but a definitive diagnosis is only made in approximately 50% of cases [21]. This method is optimal particularly in distal obstruction as Bismuth I and II. A technical success rate of 66.7% and a clinical success of 86.7% were found in a multicenter clinical trial [19]. The internal drainage by EBD is the less invasive technique and the most comfortable for the patient [14].

The endoscopic nasobiliary drainage was introduced at the beginning of the 1980s with similar advantages and complications. The availability of an external drain allows contrast cholangiography at any time via the nasobiliary tube and permits evaluation of the volume and color biliary secretions [20]. Success rates of the initial procedure ranged from 24 to 78%. Although the discomfort of the patient is imposed by nasal drainage, endoscopic nasobiliary drainage is a better way to improve the durability and reduce cholangitis than endobiliary stenting [3].

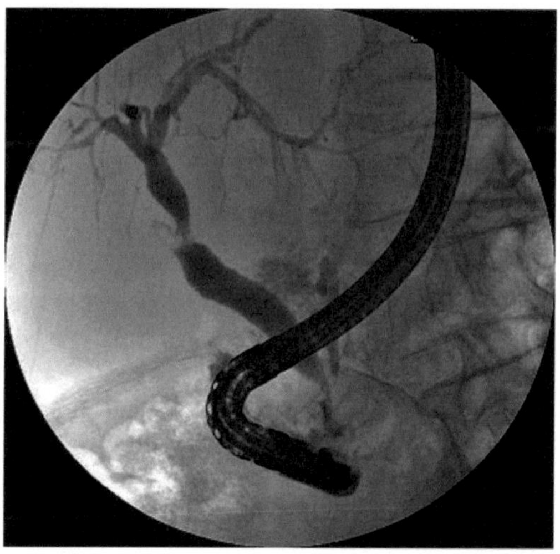

Figure 1.
ERCP.

2.3 Complications

One of the major disadvantages of an endoscopic approach is the contamination of the sterile environment of the biliary tree; this can lead to severe cholangitis and biliary sepsis. Other complications that have been reported include pancreatitis, duodenal perforation, post-sphincterotomy bleeding, biliary perforation, and tube occlusion. The morbidity reported rates are of 44.3% for the endoscopy biliary drainage [15]. Cholangitis is reported in 27–33% of the patients. The initial technical failure rate is reported in 16–21.5% of the drainages, and the rate of conversion to other procedures is of 26.5%. The pancreatitis is reported in 9% of the procedures [5, 15]. The retroperitoneal or duodenal perforation is only presented in 2% of the patients and bleeding in 1% [5].

3. Percutaneous biliary drainage

Interventionism is defined as the practice of diagnostic and therapeutic procedures through minimal incisions, performed with catheters, guides, balloons, and stents and controlled and guided by fluoroscopy, ultrasound, computed tomography, or magnetic resonance. The application of percutaneous biliary tract has been, for at least a decade, an advance in the management of seriously ill patients, which are sometimes inoperable [14, 22].

3.1 Types of drainage

Depending on the drainage site, these can be classified into three types [23]:

- Internal: the prosthesis used in the obstruction point communicating the segment prestenotic with poststenotic. The drainage is always toward the interior of the duodenum (**Figure 2**).
- External: the catheter lodged above the obstruction, the drainage of the bile, is always outward (**Figure 3**).
- Internal/external: the distal end of the catheter with orifices is placed in the duodenum; if the external drainage is open, the bile will leak to the outside, and if it is closed it will drain to the duodenum like an internal drainage (**Figure 4**).

3.1 Technique

The procedure is performed with conscious sedation. Pre-procedural planning should involve evaluation and extension of the exact level and extension of the stenosis and selection of the most appropriate liver segments for drainage and assessment of an appropriate access route, mostly by ultrasound guidance. This is particularly important when segmental bile duct obstruction is suspected, and every attempt should be made to avoid contaminating regions of the biliary tree that will not be drained (**Figure 5**).

Biliary drainage is most often performed using fluoroscopic guidance, after initial puncture of a bile duct using ultrasound guidance. There is no consensus as to whether stents should be placed from the hilum all the way down to the common bile duct through the papilla of Vater in the duodenum. Although many authors advocate stenting through the papilla in distal obstructions, there is no evidence

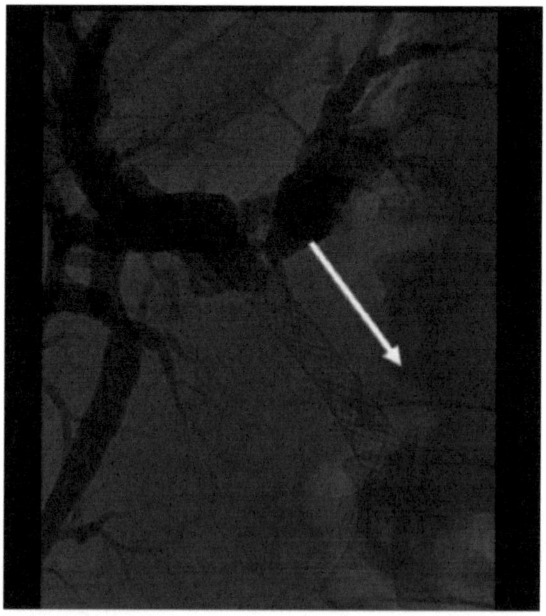

Figure 2.
Internal drainage of the bile duct.

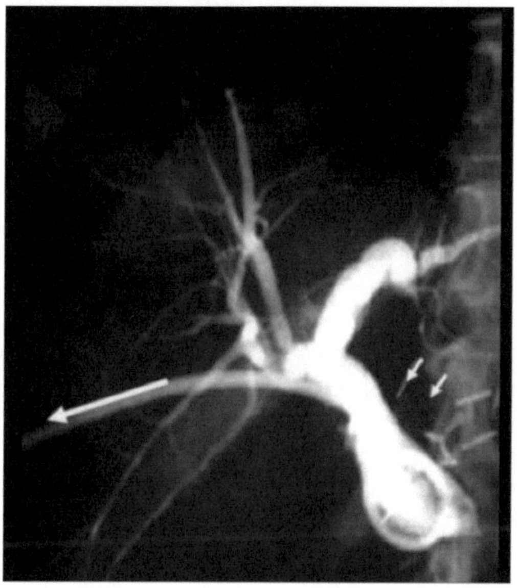

Figure 3.
External drainage of the bile duct.

that this improves patency in proximal bile duct strictures. As hilar cholangiocarcinomas are often very rigid, it may in some cases be useful to pre-dilate the stricture to facilitate the insertion of a stent.

Self-expanding metal stents are preferred because they have higher patency rates, lower overall cost, and less hospital stay than plastic stents. Metallic stents have thermal memory and expand to their maximum width when they reach body temperature, which usually occurs in 24–48 hours. If the expansion is not adequate after 28 hours, dilatation of the stent with balloon catheter may be necessary for successful drainage [24, 25].

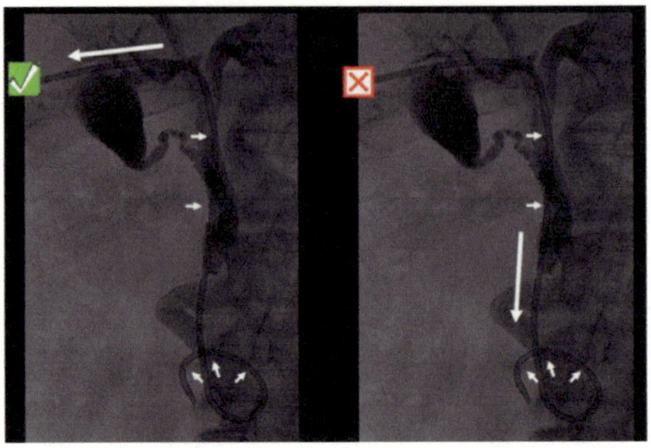

Figure 4.
Internal/external drainage.

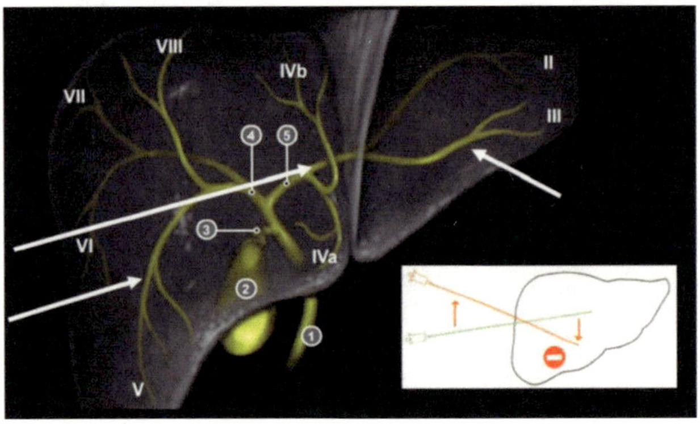

Figure 5.
Puncture external access to the biliary tree.

3.2 Advantages

The PTBD is associated with higher rates of successful biliary drainage and lower rates of cholangitis. Also, it has a distinct advantage over ERCP in that with ultrasound guidance, one or more appropriate segments for drainage can be chosen and injection of contrast medium in segments that are too small to be drained can be prevented. This is the method of drainage of the bile duct in patients with cholangiocarcinoma Bismuth types III and IV. And it is the method for election if the endoscopic drainage presented failure. This technique presents only a 5% conversion rate compared with 26.5% for EBD. The incidence of pancreatitis after PTBD has been reported in 0% compared with the 9% for EBD [15, 19, 26].

3.3 Complications

The incidence of PCT with metal stents varies from 8 to 42% complications which can be classified into early (occurring within 30 days) and late. Early complications, with exception of pain, are observed in approximately 25% to 50% of patients. Of which approximately a half were related to the procedure. These include: pain at te puncture site, bile leak with risk of biliary peritonitis and formation of biloma, hemorrage that includes hemobilia, biliovenous fistula, arterial injury, cholangitis and septicemia, acute pancreatitis, and problems related to the cateter such as sprain or dislocation.

The punctures of the right lobe are painful since the needle has to cross the intercostal space. The left lobe punctures are associated with an increased risk of bile loss and, therefore, biliary peritonitis that can cause an acute abdomen. The punctures on the right side are also associated with the risk of pneumothorax and hemothorax.

Hemorrhage usually resolves spontaneously; if persistent, a CT angiogram should be performed, and if it shows extravasation of active contrast or pseudoaneurysm, it is necessary to perform an embolization. The biliovenous fistulae present with hemorrhage in the catheter or hemobilia and can be diagnosed with cholangiography with a filling of venous vascular radicles or portal hepatic radicles. They can be managed by temporarily holding the catheter or by changing the catheter to a larger orifice catheter.

The occlusion of the stent may be due to tumor growth, excessive tumor growth, or mud. Recurrent cholangitis due to stent occlusion is observed in approximately 30% of cases, which requires repeat stenting [1, 13, 24].

4. Conclusion

There are certain advantages to both PTBD and EBD. In clinical practice, it is recommended to choose PTBD or EBD, depending on the location of the obstruction, the purpose of drainage (as a preoperative procedure or palliative treatment), and the level of experience in biliary drainage in hospital centers, so it is of great importance to individualize each case and in case of initial failure to perform the conversion of the procedure with the purpose of improving the prognosis of patients with cholangiocarcinoma.

Conflict of interest

We have no conflict of interests.

Acronyms and abbreviations

PBD	preoperative biliary drainage
EBD	endoscopic biliary drainage
PTBD	percutaneous biliary drainage
ERCP	endoscopic retrograde cholangiopancreatography
ENBD	endoscopic nasobiliary drainage

Author details

Gómez-Torres Gustavo Ángel* and Hernández-García Fernando Santiago
Hospital Civil de Guadalajara "Dr. Juan I. Menchaca", Guadalajara, Mexico

*Address all correspondence to: gustavo_angel57@hotmail.com

References

[1] Shim DJ, Gwon DI, Han K, Kim Y, Ko G-Y, Shin JH, et al. Percutaneous metallic stent placement for palliative management of malignant biliary hilar obstruction. Korean Journal of Radiology. 2018;**19**(4):597

[2] Moole H, Bechtold M, Puli SR. Efficacy of preoperative biliary drainage in malignant obstructive jaundice: A meta-analysis and systematic review. World journal of surgical oncology. 2016;**14**(1):182. Available from: http://wjso.biomedcentral.com/articles/10.1186/s12957-016-0933-2

[3] Liu J, Wu J, Wang J, Shu G, Wang Y, Lou C, et al. Endoscopic biliary drainage versus percutaneous transhepatic biliary drainage in patients with resectable hilar cholangiocarcinoma: A systematic review and meta-analysis. Journal of Laparoendoscopic & Advanced Surgical Techniques. Part A. 2018;**28**(9):1053-1060

[4] Van Heek NT, Busch OR, Van Gulik TM, Gouma DJ. Preoperative biliary drainage for pancreatic cancer. Minerva Medica. 2014;**105**(2):99-107

[5] Hameed A, Pang T, Chiou J, Pleass H, Lam V, Hollands M, et al. Percutaneous vs. endoscopic pre-operative biliary drainage in hilar cholangiocarcinoma: A systematic review and meta-analysis. HPB. 2016;**18**(5):400-410

[6] Soares KC, Kamel I, Cosgrove DP, Herman JM, Pawlik TM. Hilar cholangiocarcinoma: Diagnosis, treatment options, and management. Hepatobiliary Surgery and Nutrition. 2014;**3**(1):18-34

[7] Xu X, Li J, Wu J, Zhu R, Ji W. A systematic review and meta-analysis of intraluminal brachytherapy versus stent alone in the treatment of malignant obstructive jaundice. Cardiovascular and Interventional Radiology. 2018;**41**(2):206-217

[8] Lu J, Guo J-H, Zhu H-D, Zhu G-Y, Wang Y, Zhang Q, et al. Palliative treatment with radiation-emitting metallic stents in unresectable Bismuth type III or IV hilar cholangiocarcinoma. ESMO Open. 2017;**2**(4):e000242

[9] Wiggers JK, Groot Koerkamp B, Cieslak KP, Doussot A, van Klaveren D, Allen PJ, et al. Postoperative mortality after liver resection for perihilar cholangiocarcinoma: Development of a risk score and importance of biliary drainage of the future liver remnant. Journal of the American College of Surgeons. 2016;**223**(2):321-331.e1

[10] Ramanathan R, Borrebach J, Tohme S, Tsung A. Preoperative biliary drainage is associated with increased complications after liver resection for proximal cholangiocarcinoma. Journal of Gastrointestinal Surgery. 2018;**22**(11):1950-1957

[11] Li M, Li K, Qi X, Wu W, Zheng L, He C, et al. Percutaneous transhepatic biliary stent implantation for obstructive jaundice of perihilar cholangiocarcinoma: A prospective study on predictors of stent patency and survival in 92 patients. Journal of Vascular and Interventional Radiology. 2016;**27**(7):1047-1055.e2

[12] Sakata J, Shirai Y, Tsuchiya Y, Wakai T, Nomura T, Hatakeyama K. Preoperative cholangitis independently increases in-hospital mortality after combined major hepatic and bile duct resection for hilar cholangiocarcinoma. Langenbeck's Archives of Surgery. 2009;**394**(6):1065-1072

[13] Ruys AT, Rauws EA, Busch ORC, Lameris JS, Gouma DJ, van Gulik TM. Preoperative biliary drainage. In: Lau WY, editor. Hilar Cholangiocarcinoma. Dordrecht, Netherlands: Springer; 2013. pp. 139-146

Available from: http://link.springer.com/10.1007/978-94-007-6473-6_13

[14] Kagedan DJ, Mosko JD, Dixon ME, Karanicolas PJ, Wei AC, Goyert N, et al. Changes in preoperative endoscopic and percutaneous bile drainage in patients with periampullary cancer undergoing pancreaticoduodenectomy in Ontario: Effect on clinical practice of a randomized trial. Current Oncology. 2018;**25**(5):e430-e435. Available from: http://current-oncology.com/index.php/oncology/article/view/4007

[15] Al Mahjoub A, Menahem B, Fohlen A, Dupont B, Alves A, Launoy G, et al. Preoperative biliary drainage in patients with resectable perihilar cholangiocarcinoma: Is percutaneous transhepatic biliary drainage safer and more effective than endoscopic biliary drainage? A meta-analysis. Journal of Vascular and Interventional Radiology. 2017;**28**(4):576-582

[16] Soehendra N, Reynders-Frederix V. Palliative bile duct drainage: A new endoscopic method of introducing a transpapillary drain. Endoscopy. 1980;**12**(01):8-11

[17] Knyrim K, Wagner HJ, Pausch J, Vakil N. A prospective, randomized, controlled trial of metal stents for malignant obstruction of the common bile duct. Endoscopy. 1993;**25**(03):207-212

[18] Stern N, Sturgess R. Endoscopic therapy in the management of malignant biliary obstruction. European Journal of Surgical Oncology. 2008;**34**(3):313-317

[19] Paik WH, Lee TH, Park DH, Choi J-H, Kim S-O, Jang S, et al. EUS-guided biliary drainage versus ERCP for the primary palliation of malignant biliary obstruction: A multicenter randomized clinical trial. The American Journal of Gastroenterology. 2018;**113**(7):987-997

[20] Kloek JJ, van der Gaag NA, Aziz Y, Rauws EAJ, van Delden OM, Lameris JS, et al. Endoscopic and percutaneous preoperative biliary drainage in patients with suspected hilar cholangiocarcinoma. Journal of Gastrointestinal Surgery. 2010;**14**(1):119-125

[21] Parsi MA, Li A, Li C, Goggins M. DNA methylation alterations in endoscopic retrograde cholangiopancreatography brush samples of patients with suspected pancreaticobiliary disease. Clinical Gastroenterology and Hepatology. 2008;**6**(11):1270-1278

[22] Inamdar S, Slattery E, Bhalla R, Sejpal DV, Trindade AJ. Comparison of adverse events for endoscopic vs percutaneous biliary drainage in the treatment of malignant biliary tract obstruction in an inpatient national cohort. JAMA Oncology. 2016;**2**(1):112

[23] Sebastián/ES D-S. Manejo de la obstrucción maligna de la vía biliar en radiología intervencionista. In: Poster presented at Seram 2012; Granada, España; 2012

[24] Inal M, Aksungur E, Akgul E, Oguz M, Seydaoglu G. Percutaneous placement of metallic stents in malignant biliary obstruction: One-stage or two-stage procedure? Pre-dilate or not? Cardiovascular and Interventional Radiology. 2003;**26**(1):40-45

[25] George C. Interventional radiology in the management of malignant biliary obstruction. World Journal of Gastrointestinal Oncology. 2010;**2**(3):146

[26] Heedman PA, Åstradsson E, Blomquist K, Sjödahl R. Palliation of malignant biliary obstruction: Adverse events are common after percutaneous transhepatic biliary drainage. Scandinavian Journal of Surgery. 2018;**107**(1):48-53

Chapter 3

Bile Duct Cancer: Preoperative Evaluation and Management

Tommaso Stecca, Bruno Pauletti, Luca Bonariol, Ezio Caratozzolo and Marco Massani

Abstract

Cholangiocarcinomas (CCAs) are malignant tumors that can develop anywhere along the biliary tree. Almost 10% of cholangiocarcinomas arise from the intrahepatic bile ducts (iCCA); 50–60% from the bifurcation of the hepatic duct (perihilar cholangiocarcinoma, pCCA); and 20–30% from the distal bile duct (dCCA). The 7th edition of the AJCC staging system, released in 2010, divides the tumors into two major categories: perihilar (pCCA) and distal (dCCA) cholangiocarcinoma, given the differences in anatomy of the bile duct and consideration of local factors related to resectability. There are separate histological classifications for intrahepatic and extrahepatic cholangiocarcinoma. The majority of CCAs (90%) are well or moderately differentiated adenocarcinomas. Other features include invasiveness with early neural, perineural, periductal and lymphatic infiltration (more than 50% of cases at diagnosis) and longitudinal subepithelial infiltration along the wall of the bile duct up to 2 cm proximally and 1 cm distally. In this chapter the extrhepatic bile duct cancers are analyzed.

Keywords: bile duct, cancer, embolization, drainage

1. Introduction

Cholangiocarcinomas (CCAs) are malignant tumors that can develop anywhere along the biliary tree [1]. Almost 10% of cholangiocarcinomas arise from the intrahepatic bile ducts (iCCA); 50–60% from the bifurcation of the hepatic duct (perihilar cholangiocarcinoma, pCCA), previously called Klatskin from the name of the author who first described it in 1965; and 20–30% from the distal bile duct (dCCA) [2]. In the previous editions of the American Joint Committee on Cancer (AJCC), staging system of extrahepatic bile duct tumors has been considered as a single entity [3]. The seventh edition of the AJCC staging system, released in 2010, divides the tumors into two major categories: perihilar cholangiocarcinoma (pCCA) and distal cholangiocarcinoma (dCCA) [4], given the differences in anatomy of the bile duct and consideration of local factors related to resectability [5]. For epidemiological findings it is advisable to avoid misclassification and to define subtypes according to the WHO classification as iCCA, pCCA, and dCCA [6–8].

There are separate histological classifications for intrahepatic and extrahepatic cholangiocarcinoma. The majority of CCAs (90%) are well- or moderately differentiated adenocarcinomas with a tendency to develop intense desmoplastic reactions due to the rapid proliferation of the tumor-associated stromal cells and cancer-associated fibroblasts. Other features include invasiveness with early neural, perineural, periductal, and lymphatic infiltration (more than 50% of cases at diagnosis) and longitudinal subepithelial infiltration along the wall of the bile duct up to 2 cm proximally and 1 cm distally [9].

Although there is little data on this neoplasm, incidence rates and mortality seem to be declining in many countries. Through analysis of the SEER database, the mortality rate in the United States fell from 0.6 to 0.3 per 100,000 and incidence rates from 1.08 to 0.82 per 100,000. These data are probably more difficult to obtain because of the common ICD classification for both gallbladder and extrahepatic CCA tumors [10].

pCCA is the most common form with variable prevalence according to geographic areas, between 46 and 97% [4, 11, 12]. pCCA is diagnosed earlier and smaller than the intrahepatic variant because of its early presentation with indolent jaundice in 90% of cases or with cholangitis in about 10%. The infiltrative periductal histotype is the most common form; the exophytic mass-forming or intraductal papillary is less frequent [13]. Distal cholangiocarcinoma (dCCA) may derive from two precursors, recognized in the last WHO classification: intraductal papillary neoplasia and biliary intraepithelial neoplasia [14]. Similar to the pCCA, patients present at the onset of cholestatic jaundice and cholangitis secondary to biliary obstruction.

The prognosis is generally poor with a 5-year survival that is less than 5%. The median survival rate for patients with the intrahepatic variant is between 18 and 30 months; however, the perihilar variant has a median between 14 and 24 months. The only curative therapeutic option can be expected from liver surgery for early-stage tumors. After surgery, the recurrence rate is between 60 and 90%. However, given that most patients come to the attention of the surgeon with an advanced stage of disease, thus precluding the surgical option, 75% of patients die 1 year after diagnosis. The main causes of death among patients are cachexia, liver failure, and sepsis due to biliary tract obstruction. Although 1-year survival increased from 16% (1975–1979) to 28% (1995–1999), the 5-year survival showed no significant change [2].

2. Preoperative biliary drainage

2.1 Obstructive jaundice

Biliary obstruction leads to numerous pathophysiological consequences both at a local level, in the biliary tree, and at a systemic one. Affected patients are at high risk of liver insufficiency, renal failure, heart failure, coagulopathy, immunodeficiency, infectious complications, and, therefore, increased morbidity and mortality [15].

2.1.1 Local effects

Pressure inside the biliary tree is normally between 5 and 10 cmH_2O, but in case of complete obstruction, it can reach 30 cmH_2O. The biliary secretion is prevented when it exceeds the value of 10 cmH_2O [16]. Cholestasis favors bacterial overgrowth of the bile which, under normal conditions, is sterile. Furthermore, biliary hypertension causes a "cholangio-venous" reflux sustained by the increased permeability of bile ductules, thus favoring bacterial translocation and finally severe infections and sepsis [17, 18], as well as periportal neutrophilic infiltrate [19].

Increased pressure in the biliary system can gradually reduce the production of bile. However, the risk of lithogenesis is low due to the greater reduction in the secretion of cholesterol and phospholipids than bile salts (which guarantee the solubility of cholesterol in the bile). When the obstruction is resolved, the restoration of cholesterol and phospholipid secretion is inversely faster than the bile salt ones, thus favoring the lithogenesis responsible for the early obstruction of biliary stents [19, 20].

2.1.2 Systemic effects

Jaundice influences liver metabolic and synthetic function. The inhibition of cytochrome P450 and the reduction of aerobic and oxidative metabolism lead to an increase in oxidative stress, cell apoptosis, and alteration of drug metabolism. The reduced liver synthetic capacity leads to a reduction in the levels of albumin, coagulation factors, and immunoglobulins [20].

The proliferation of the intestinal microbial flora is favored by the interruption of the recirculation of the bile salts and is associated with the dysfunction of the intestinal mucosal barrier and the bacterial translocation with consequent increase in the absorption of endotoxins hereby produced [19]. Increased intestinal permeability also plays a key role in the development of a potential septic state and renal complications [21].

Endotoxin (lipopolysaccharide) is usually inactivated by the hepatic reticuloendothelial system, but organ dysfunction—associated with increased endogenous production—leads to a systemic inflammatory response syndrome (SIRS) that may result in the multi-organ dysfunction syndrome (hemodynamic instability and renal failure) [22–25].

Acute renal failure occurs in 10% of jaundiced patients. This complication is associated with high mortality (70–80%). In addition, endotoxinemia stimulates the secretion of vasoactive prostaglandins and cytokines that are responsible for tubular necrosis and fibrin deposition with further reduction of glomerular filtration [26–28].

The alteration of the immune system and the septic manifestations are mainly due to the insufficiency of the cellular immunity (T lymphocytes) induced by the release of cytokines (TNFα, IL-1, IL-6, IFNγ), prostaglandins, and other mediators of inflammation [29–31].

The hemorrhagic diathesis is due to coagulation disorders induced by both complement activation and reduced hepatic prothrombin and other vitamin K-dependent factors (VII, IX, X, C-S-Z protein synthesis). The absence of bile salts in the intestine prevents the absorption of vitamin K [32].

2.2 Guidelines

2.2.1 Perihilar cholangiocarcinoma

In patients with perihilar cholangiocarcinoma and jaundice, the National Comprehensive Cancer Network (NCCN) guidelines recommend to consider preoperative biliary drainage. The decision should be always made by a multidisciplinary team at an HPB center. The different expertise of the different centers significantly affects the choice between the endoscopic and the percutaneous approach. Bile drainage can be performed either endoscopically or percutaneously. There are currently no randomized clinical trials comparing these two types of drainage. Most retrospective studies have not shown any significant differences, both in terms of bilirubinemia reduction and complications [33]. The effectiveness of preoperative biliary drainage was analyzed by Farges et al. [34] in a multicenter retrospective study performed on 366 patients who underwent pCCA resection between 1997 and 2008 with right or left hepatectomy without resection of the pancreatic head. One hundred and eighty patients (180/366; 49.1%) received biliary drain placement. Although drainage did not result in a significant change in postoperative mortality, a subanalysis showed a decrease in normalized postoperative mortality for preoperative bilirubin in patients undergoing right hepatectomy (adjusted OR = 0.29; CI 0.11–0.77; p = 0.013) and an increase in postoperative mortality in patients undergoing left hepatectomy (OR = 4.06 CI 1.01–16.3; p = 0.035). In particular, the cause of major postoperative mortality in the right hepatectomy group was liver failure and sepsis in the left hepatectomy group. Endoscopic nasobiliary drainage seems to be the most appropriate method of PBD in terms of minimizing the risks of tract seeding and inflammatory reactions [33].

2.2.2 Distal cholangiocarcinoma

The latest guidelines issued by the NCCN for the endoscopic treatment of biliary obstruction in dCCA recommend different treatments based on clinical status (**Table 1**) [35].

One of the reasons for greater debate concerns the balance between risks and benefits in the preoperative stenting of neoplastic biliary obstruction in resectable patients. The meta-analyses that investigated this topic concluded that preoperative biliary drainage should not be performed routinely, given the absence of difference in mortality but, above all, the increased associated morbidity [36–39]. However, stenting is recommended in patients with cholangitis, pruritus, coagulopathy, and renal failure or for whom surgical treatment is delayed for at least 1 week [35]. The scientific debate is also open regarding the type of stent, plastic or metal (partially or completely coated). It has been shown that coated metal stents have a lower dislocation rate and a longer patency time [40]. On the other hand, plastic stents are easier to position or replace and have an advantageous cost-benefit profile. However, a recent meta-analysis has shown that in patients with an overall survival of more than 6 months, the placement of the metal stent is associated with a better cost-benefit and quality of life [41]. Patency duration, morbidity, mortality, and repositioning rates were investigated in other studies [42–45] that demonstrated the superiority of the metal stent (short intrapancreatic or coated) due to increased patency resulting in a reduced need for additional endoscopy. The guidelines compiled by the NCCN and the European Society of Gastrointestinal Endoscopy (ESGE) indicate as a first choice the plastic stent in patients diagnosed with uncertain malignancy and those with an unfavorable prognosis (≤3 months according to NCCN; ≤4 months according to ESGE) [35, 46].

Status	Recommendation
Resectable tumor, jaundice	Preoperative biliary drainage only in symptomatic patients (cholangitis, fever, pruritus, sepsis, coagulopathy, renal failure) or in which the surgical program is delayed by at least 1 week Plastic or metal stent (if diagnosis histologically confirmed)
"Borderline resectable" tumor, candidate for neoadjuvant therapy, jaundice	Self-expanding metal stent
Unresectable tumor, intraoperative finding, jaundice	Self-expanding metal stent if no surgical bypass is performed during surgery
Metastatic tumor, jaundice	Self-expanding metal stent*

**Many members of the NCCN panel point to the plastic stent in patients with a life expectancy of less than 3 months.*

Table 1.
Neoplastic biliary obstruction. NCCN endoscopic treatment guidelines.

3. Liver function tests

pCCA surgical approach may also require extended liver resection. The hepatic parenchyma must be removed, but also the residual volume and its ability to guarantee acceptable residual liver function must be carefully assessed [47]. In 2011 the International Study Group of Liver Surgery published and updated the posthepatectomy liver failure definition and grading [48]. Posthepatectomy liver failure (PHLF) has been defined as an "acquired deterioration in the ability of the liver to maintain its synthetic, excretory and detoxifying functions, characterized by an increased INR, and hyperbilirubinemia on or after postoperative day 5." PHLF is then differentiated into three grades (A, B, and C) based on clinical and invasive management [48]. The presence of liver disease and liver function correlates with the critical residual liver volume able to predict PHLF. The limit for a safe resection ranges from 20 to 30% future remnant liver among patients with normal liver function. However, this limit must be raised to over 40% in case of risk factors related to patient, liver, or surgery [47].

3.1 Volumetry

Computed tomography and magnetic resonance imaging are used increasingly to measure liver volume in patients evaluated for resection. Numerous factors can influence the accuracy of preoperative liver volumetry: the phase of contrast administration, slice thickness, use of CT versus MRI, varying image processing software, and inter-user variability, as well as the degree to which non-parenchymal structures are erroneously included within the functional liver volume [49].

In 2002 Vauthey published the formula to estimate total liver volume (TLV) based on body surface area (BSA). The formula obtained was TLV = 794.41 + 1267.28 × BSA (m^2), and a formula based on patient weight also was derived: TLV = 191.80 + 18.51 × weight (kg) [50].

In 2015 Martel compared the two techniques, the measured and the estimated liver volume, to determine the accuracy and variability of each volumetric method [49]. The conclusion of his study is that TLV is best evaluated by direct radiologic measurement rather than by indirect estimation. Indeed, estimated volumetry leads to a clinically significant over- or underestimation of the future liver remnant (≥5% in 31.9% of patients) and is more frequently associated with an underestimation of the estimated TLV and an overestimation of the estimated remnant future liver ratio [49].

3.2 Indocyanine green clearance test

Many quantitative liver function tests have been proposed, but they are impractical in a clinical setting because of excessive cost, need for multiple samples and prolonged catheterization, and risk of allergic reaction. Indocyanine green (ICG) clearance test is considered the most predictive test of operative mortality after hepatectomy if compared to other tests such as the amino acid clearance test or aminopyrine breath test [51]. The indocyanine green dye is absorbed by the hepatocytes and excreted via the biliary tract without enterohepatic recirculation. The percentage of retention can be measured by pulsed spectrophotometry using an optical sensor [52]. The $ICGR_{15}$ describes the percentage of circulatory retention of indocyanine green during the first 15 min after bolus injection. The cutoff value of ICG retention normal value in healthy patients is between 8 and 15%, and the cutoff value that allows a major hepatectomy is between 14 and 17% [53, 54]. Minor resections may be performed for values that reach 22% and limited hepatectomies (bisegmentectomies) to values up to 40%. Some authors claim that laparoscopic limited wedge resections could be tolerated for values even greater [55]. Bilirubin and indocyanine green bind to the same carrier in the transport phase in hepatocytes, determining a competitive inhibition. For that reason, ICG retention is not valid in jaundiced patients.

4. Portal vein embolization

Portal vein embolization (PVE) is indicated in patients in whom a major resection or a parenchymal resection of more than 50–60% of the TLV is programmed, with the goal to prevent or reduce the risk of posthepatectomy liver failure [Benson 2014]. Although there are no randomized trials comparing the operative risk in patients subjected or not to PVE, a reduction in mortality is demonstrated from the retrospective series present in the literature in up to 0–2% of patients resected after PVE [Benson 2014]. In contrast, mortality rates vary between 10 and 21% in HPB centers where the indication to the PVE has been given with a residual liver volume less than 25–30%.

5. Preoperative staging systems

5.1 Perihilar cholangiocarcinoma

The Bismuth-Corlette classification is the most used to program the best derivative approach because it evaluates the longitudinal tumor extension. Four types of pCCA are distinguished based on their perihilar extension: type I, tumor confined to the common hepatic duct; type II, tumor limited to the confluence of the hepatic duct, without involvement of the second-order ducts; type III, tumor involving the confluence with extension to the right (IIIA) or left (IIIB) hepatic duct; and type IV, tumor affecting the biliary confluence with the involvement of secondary intrahepatic ducts on both sides. This system is used to plan the surgical treatment, from the resection (type I and II) to a major hepatectomy (type III). Type IV is traditionally considered nonsurgical, except for liver transplantation [56], but recently, curative surgery has also been attempted in type IV tumors that extend backward for less than 2 cm from the hilum. However, the Bismuth-Corlette classification system lacks important resectability information such as vascular infiltration, local or distant lymph node metastatic spread, and lobar hepatic atrophy, and therefore this system has no prognostic value and does not correlate with survival results [57, 58]. Moreover, in some cases, a precise Bismuth-Corlette classification can be difficult to define at the imaging due to the poor definition of the longitudinal extension in case of subepithelial infiltration (infiltrative forms) or of mucosal diffusion (papillary polypoid forms) [13].

The classification proposed by the Memorial Sloan-Kettering Cancer Center (MSKCC) details three factors related to tumor extension: the position and extent of biliary involvement (similar to the Bismuth-Corlette classification), portal vein invasion, and hepatic lobar atrophy, independently of lymph node or distant metastases. It is used for the selection of patients fit for surgery [59].

In the seventh edition of the AJCC/UICC staging system, the pCCA was staged as a separate entity based on anatomo-pathological staging (pathological TNM). The AJCC system also considers involvement of the portal vein and hepatic artery, lymph node status, and distant metastases. It is mainly used as a postoperative staging system and has a minimal utility to assess the resectability. An initial stage tumor (T1) is limited to the bile duct wall. T2 tumors extend beyond the bile duct wall, invading the periductal fat (T2a) or liver (T2b), and often present as periductal infiltrative forms or as a nodular mass showing irregular duct wall thickening with contrast enhancement. The T3 stage includes locally invasive lesions involving the liver, gallbladder, pancreas, or ipsilateral portal vein or hepatic artery. The T4 stage includes widely invasive tumors, with bilateral extension to the portal vein or to the main portal trunk, the common hepatic artery, the contralateral vascular extension, and the involvement of the second-order bile ducts or to adjacent organs (colon, stomach, duodenum, or abdominal wall). The involvement of the hepatic parenchyma is classified as T2 instead of T3 since parenchymal involvement alone has a better prognosis than unilateral vascular involvement.

Numerous experiences have shown inaccuracies offered by the AJCC system, which may, in part, be due to not having taken into account the depth of the tumor invasion [60]. Given the limitations of the various staging systems and the difficulty in comparing the results in various centers, DeOliveira and an international panel of experts have introduced a new staging system for the pCCA, which also includes new factors to improve and standardize the determination of prognosis and tumor reporting [61]. This new system is derived from the Bismuth-Corlette classification for the evaluation of the involvement of the biliary tree but also considers (a) the size of the tumor (diameter >1 cm, 1–3 cm, or ≥3 cm); (b) tumor morphology, periductal or nodular-sclerosing or mass-forming, intraductal or polypoid, and mixed; (c) degree and position of the hepatic artery infiltration and of the portal vein encasement; (d) hepatic lobar atrophy and future liver remnant volume; (e) other liver diseases (fibrosis, nonalcoholic steatohepatitis, or PSC); (f) lymph nodes; and (g) distant metastases, including the liver and peritoneal ones. Therefore, this staging is applicable in the preoperative setting and includes well-established prognostic factors. The inclusion of the type of macroscopic tumor growth has never been included in other staging systems and has been shown to be a predictor of survival [62]. However, this staging system is rather complicated and also includes some prognostic factors not yet validated, such as tumor size, lobar atrophy, and the volumetric analysis [59]. The validity of this new system still needs verification in large prospective studies.

5.2 Distal cholangiocarcinoma

The first classification system that has assigned a definition for the dCCA separated from the pCCA is the seventh edition of the AJCC/UICC classification. This has been an important step because the differences between the two extrahepatic forms have been recognized. For example, the depth of ductal invasion and pancreatic invasion is significantly more common in dCCA [63]. Indeed, depth of invasion, lymph node metastasis, perineural and microscopic vascular invasion as well as the invasion of the pancreas, and the R0 resection are significant survival predictors [64, 65]. The pattern of lymph node metastasis differs between the three types of CCA and is most commonly observed in the dCCA [66]. Several studies have suggested that the number of pathological lymph nodes is an independent prognostic factor; more than two metastatic lymph nodes are predictive of a worse prognosis. In the AJCC classification, the T stage distinguishes T1 and T2 tumors based on the microscopic tumor growth pattern if confined to the bile duct or beyond it. The TNM staging system shares some of the features of the pCCA: T1 and T2 tumors are confined to the bile duct wall (T1) or invade the bile duct without invasion to adjacent organs (T2). Invasion of adjacent organs (pancreas, stomach, and duodenum) is considered T3. The invasion of the celiac tripod and superior mesenteric artery is considered T4. Moreover, the TNM classification presents similarities with that of pancreatic cancer. The lymph node staging has two stages (N0 and N1). Unlike proximal tumors, lymph node staging is performed at the time of surgery with the sampling of at least 12 lymph nodes.

Author details

Tommaso Stecca, Bruno Pauletti, Luca Bonariol, Ezio Caratozzolo and Marco Massani*
Surgical Department, Hepato-Pancreato-Biliary Regional Referral Center, AULSS2 Marca Trevigiana - Treviso Regional Hospital, Italy

*Address all correspondence to: marco.massani@aulss2.veneto.it

References

[1] Razumilava N, Gores GJ. Cholangiocarcinoma. Lancet. 2014;**383**:2168-2179. DOI: 10.1016/S0140-6736(13)61903-0

[2] Mosconi S, Beretta GD, Labianca R, Zampino MG, Gatta G, et al. Cholangiocarcinoma. Critical Reviews in Oncology/Hematology. 2009;**69**:259-270. DOI: 10.1016/j.critrevonc.2008.09.008

[3] Greene FL, AJC on C and ACS. AJCC Cancer Staging Manual. 6th ed. New York: Springer-Verlag; 2002. pp. 255-281

[4] Edge S, Byrd DR, Compton CC, Fritz AG, Greene FL, Trotti A. AJCC Cancer Staging Manual. 7th ed. New York, NY: Springer. DOI: 10.1007/978-1-4757-3656-4. Epub ahead of print 2009

[5] Nakanuma Y, Kakuda Y. Pathologic classification of cholangiocarcinoma: New concepts. Best Practice & Research. Clinical Gastroenterology. 2015;**29**: 277-293. DOI: 10.1016/j.bpg.2015.02.006

[6] Blechacz B, Komuta M, Roskams T, Gores GJ. Clinical diagnosis and staging of cholangiocarcinoma. Nature Reviews. Gastroenterology & Hepatology. 2011;**8**:512-522. DOI: 10.1038/nrgastro.2011.131

[7] Bridgewater J, Galle PR, Khan SA, Llovet JM, Park J-W, et al. Guidelines for the diagnosis and management of intrahepatic cholangiocarcinoma. Journal of Hepatology. 2014;**60**:1268-1289. DOI: 10.1016/j.jhep.2014.01.021

[8] DeOliveira ML, Cunningham SC, Cameron JL, Kamangar F, Winter JM, et al. Cholangiocarcinoma: Thirty-one-year experience with 564 patients at a single institution. Annals of Surgery. 2007;**245**:755-762. DOI: 10.1097/01.sla.0000251366.62632.d3

[9] Cadamuro M, Stecca T, Brivio S, Mariotti V, Fiorotto R, et al. The deleterious interplay between tumor epithelia and stroma in cholangiocarcinoma. Biochimica et Biophysica Acta—Molecular Basis of Disease. Apr 2018;**1864**(4 Pt B):1435-1443. DOI: 10.1016/j.bbadis.2017.07.028

[10] Khan SA, Thomas HC, Davidson BR, Taylor-Robinson SD. Cholangiocarcinoma. Lancet. 8 Oct 2005;**366**(9493):1303-1314. DOI: 10.1016/S0140-6736(05)67530-7

[11] National Comprehensive Cancer Network. Hepatobiliary cancers (version 3.2018). 2018. Retrieved from: https://www.nccn.org/professionals/physician_gls/pdf/hepatobiliary.pdf [Accessed August, 29 2018

[12] Liau JY, Tsai JH, Yuan RH, Chang CN, Lee HJ, et al. Morphological subclassification of intrahepatic cholangiocarcinoma: Etiological, clinicopathological, and molecular features. Modern Pathology. 2014;**27**:1163-1173. DOI: 10.1038/modpathol.2013.241

[13] Chung YE, Kim M-J, Park YN, Choi J-Y, Pyo JY, et al. Varying appearances of cholangiocarcinoma: Radiologic-pathologic correlation. Radiographics. 2009;**29**:683-700. DOI: 10.1148/rg.293085729

[14] Nakanuma Y, Sato Y, Harada K, Sasaki M, Xu J, et al. Pathological classification of intrahepatic cholangiocarcinoma based on a new concept. World Journal of Hepatology. 2010;**2**:419-427. DOI: 10.4254/wjh.v2.i12.419

[15] Pavlidis ET, Pavlidis TE. Pathophysiological consequences of obstructive jaundice and perioperative management. Hepatobiliary & Pancreatic Diseases International.

2018;**17**:17-21. DOI: 10.1016/j.hbpd.2018.01.008

[16] Briggs CD, Peterson M. Investigation and management of obstructive jaundice. Surgery. 2007;**25**:74-80. DOI: 10.1016/j.mpsur.2007.01.005

[17] Kinney TP. Management of ascending cholangitis. Gastrointestinal Endoscopy Clinics of North America. 2007;**17**:289-306. DOI: 10.1016/j.giec.2007.03.006

[18] Kimura Y, Takada T, Kawarada Y, Nimura Y, Hirata K, et al. Definitions, pathophysiology, and epidemiology of acute cholangitis and cholecystitis: Tokyo guidelines. Journal of Hepato-Biliary-Pancreatic Surgery. 2007;**14**: 15-26. DOI: 10.1007/s00534-006-1152-y

[19] Ramappa V, Aithal GP. Jaundice: Applying lessons from physiology. Surgery (United Kingdom). 2014;**32**:627-634. DOI: 10.1016/j.mpsur.2014.09.010

[20] Fukushima S, Okuno H, Shibatani N, Nakahashi Y, Seki T, et al. Effect of biliary obstruction and internal biliary drainage on hepatic cytochrome P450 isozymes in rats. World Journal of Gastroenterology. 2008;**14**:2556-2560. DOI: 10.3748/wjg.14.2556

[21] Assimakopulos SF, Scopa CD, Vagianos C. Pathophysiology of increased permeability in obstructive jaundice. World Journal of Gastroenterology. 2007;**13**:6455-6618

[22] Koutelidakis I, Papaziogas B, Giamarellos-Bourboulis EJ, Makris J, Pavlidis T, et al. Systemic endotoxaemia following obstructive jaundice: The role of lactulose. The Journal of Surgical Research. 2003;**113**:243-247. DOI: 10.1016/S0022-4804(03)00209-9

[23] Deitch EA, Sittig K, Li M, Berg R, Specian RD. Obstructive jaundice promotes bacterial translocation from the gut. American Journal of Surgery. 1990;**159**:79-84. DOI: 10.1016/S0002-9610(05)80610-5

[24] Scott-Conner CEH, Grogan JB. The pathophysiology of biliary obstruction and its effect on phagocytic and immune function. Journal of Surgical Research. 1994;**57**:316-336. DOI: 10.1006/jsre.1994.1151

[25] Naranjo A, Cruz A, López P, Chicano M, Martín-Malo A, et al. Renal function after dopamine and fluid administration in patients with malignant obstructive jaundice. A prospective randomized study. Journal of Gastrointestinal and Liver Diseases. 2011;**20**:161-167

[26] Fogarty BJ, Parks RW, Rowlands BJ, Diamond T. Renal dysfunction in obstructive jaundice. The British Journal of Surgery. Jul 1995;**82**(7):877-884. DOI: 10.1002/bjs.1800820707. Epub ahead of print 1995

[27] Pain JA, Cahill CJ, Gilbert JM, Johnson CD, Trapnell JE, et al. Prevention of postoperative renal dysfunction in patients with obstructive jaundice: A multicentre study of bile salts and lactulose. The British Journal of Surgery. 1991;**78**:467-469

[28] Uslu A, Cayci M, Nart A, Karaca C, Zalluhoglu N, et al. Renal failure in obstructive jaundice. Hepato-Gastroenterology. 2005;**52**:52-54

[29] Nehéz L, Andersson R. Compromise of immune function in obstructive jaundice. European Journal of Surgery. 2002;**168**:315-328. DOI: 10.1080/11024150260284815

[30] Parlesak A, Schaeckeler S, Moser L, Bode C. Conjugated primary bile salts reduce permeability of endotoxin through intestinal epithelial cells and synergize with phosphatidylcholine in suppression of inflammatory cytokine

production. Critical Care Medicine. 2007;**35**:2367-2374. DOI: 10.1097/01.CCM.0000284586.84952.FB

[31] Kimmings AN, Van Deventer SJH, Obertop H, Rauws EAJ, Gouma DJ. Inflammatory and immunologic effects of obstructive jaundice: Pathogenesis and treatment. Journal of the American College of Surgeons. 1995;**181**:567-581

[32] Hunt DR, Allison MEM, Prentice CRM, Blumgart LH. Endotoxemia, disturbance of coagulation, and obstructive jaundice. American Journal of Surgery. 1982;**144**:325-329. DOI: 10.1016/0002-9610(82)90011-3

[33] Kawakami H, Kuwatani M, Onodera M, Haba S, Eto K, et al. Endoscopic nasobiliary drainage is the most suitable preoperative biliary drainage method in the management of patients with hilar cholangiocarcinoma. Journal of Gastroenterology. 2011;**46**:242-248. DOI: 10.1007/s00535-010-0298-1

[34] Farges O, Regimbeau JM, Fuks D, Le Treut YP, Cherqui D, et al. Multicentre european study of preoperative biliary drainage for hilar cholangiocarcinoma. The British Journal of Surgery. 2013;**100**:274-283. DOI: 10.1002/bjs.8950

[35] Tempero MA, Malafa MP, Al-Hawary M, Asbun H, Bain A, et al. Pancreatic adenocarcinoma, version 2.2017, NCCN clinical practice guidelines in oncology. Journal of the National Comprehensive Cancer Network. 2017;**15**:1028-1061. DOI: 10.6004/jnccn.2017.0131

[36] Sewnath ME, Karsten TM, Prins MH, Rauws EJA, Obertop H, et al. A meta-analysis on the efficacy of preoperative biliary drainage for tumors causing obstructive jaundice. Annals of Surgery. 2002;**236**:17-27. DOI: 10.1097/00000658-200207000-00005

[37] Fang Y, Wang Q, Ks G, Lin H, Xie X, et al. Preoperative biliary drainage for obstructive jaundice (review). Cochrane Database of Systematic Reviews. 12 Sep 2012;(9):1-42. DOI: 10.1002/14651858.CD005444.pub3

[38] Chen Y, Ou G, Lian G, Luo H, Huang K, et al. Effect of preoperative biliary drainage on complications following pancreatoduodenectomy: A meta-analysis. Medicine (Baltimore). 2015;**94**:e1199. DOI: 10.1097/MD.0000000000001199

[39] Scheufele F, Schorn S, Demir IE, Sargut M, Tieftrunk E, et al. Preoperative biliary stenting versus operation first in jaundiced patients due to malignant lesions in the pancreatic head: A meta-analysis of current literature. Surgery (United States). 2017;**161**:939-950. DOI: 10.1016/j.surg.2016.11.001

[40] Soderlund C, Linder S. Covered metal versus plastic stents for malignant common bile duct stenosis: A prospective, randomized, controlled trial. Gastrointestinal Endoscopy. 2006;**63**:986-995. DOI: 10.1016/j.gie.2005.11.052

[41] Martinez JM, Anene A, Bentley TGK, Cangelosi MJ, Meckley LM, et al. Cost effectiveness of metal stents in relieving obstructive jaundice in patients with pancreatic cancer. Journal of Gastrointestinal Cancer. 2017;**48**:58-65. DOI: 10.1007/s12029-016-9907-4

[42] Moss AC, Morris E, Leyden J, MacMathuna P. Malignant distal biliary obstruction: A systematic review and meta-analysis of endoscopic and surgical bypass results. Cancer Treatment Reviews. 2007;**33**:213-221. DOI: 10.1016/j.ctrv.2006.10.006

[43] Moss AC, Morris E, Mac Mathuna P. Palliative biliary stents for obstructing pancreatic carcinoma. The Cochrane Database of Systematic Reviews.

Published by John Wiley & Sons Ltd.; 2006;(1):1-11. Article No: CD004200. DOI: 0.1002/14651858.CD004200.pub2

[44] Sawas T, Al Halabi S, Parsi MA, Vargo JJ. Self-expandable metal stents versus plastic stents for malignant biliary obstruction: A meta-analysis. Gastrointestinal Endoscopy. 2015;**82**:256-267.e7. DOI: 10.1016/j.gie.2015.03.1980

[45] Olsson G, Frozanpor F, Lundell L, Enochsson L, Ansorge C, et al. Preoperative biliary drainage by plastic or self-expandable metal stents in patients with periampullary tumors: Results of a randomized clinical study. Endoscopy International Open. 2017;**5**:E798-E808. DOI: 10.1055/s-0043-110565

[46] Dumonceau JM, Tringali A, Blero D, Devière J, Laugiers R, et al. Biliary stenting: Indications, choice of stents and results: European Society of Gastrointestinal Endoscopy (ESGE) clinical guideline. Endoscopy. 2012;**44**:277-298. DOI: 10.1055/s-0031-1291633

[47] Guglielmi A, Ruzzenente A, Conci S, Valdegamberi A, Iacono C. How much remnant is enough in liver resection? Digestive Surgery. 2012;**29**:6-17. DOI: 10.1159/000335713

[48] Dematteo RP, Weitz J, Christophi C, Hugh TJ, Maddern G, et al. Posthepatectomy liver failure: A definition and grading by the international study Group of Liver Surgery (ISGLS). Surgery. 2011;**149**: 713-724. DOI: 10.1016/j.surg.2010.10.001

[49] Martel G, Cieslak KP, Huang R, Van Lienden KP, Wiggers JK, et al. Comparison of techniques for volumetric analysis of the future liver remnant: Implications for major hepatic resections. HPB. 2015;**17**:1051-1057. DOI: 10.1111/hpb.12480

[50] Vauthey JN, Abdalla EK, Doherty DA, Gertsch P, Fenstermacher MJ, et al. Body surface area and body weight predict total liver volume in western adults. Liver Transplantation. 2002;**8**:233-240. DOI: 10.1053/jlts.2002.31654

[51] Morris-Stiff G, Gomez D, Prasad R. Quantitative assessment of hepatic function and its relevance to the liver surgeon. Journal of Gastrointestinal Surgery. 2009;**13**:374-385. DOI: 10.1007/s11605-008-0564-1

[52] Akita H, Sasaki Y, Yamada T, Gotoh K, Ohigashi H, et al. Real-time intraoperative assessment of residual liver functional reserve using pulse dye densitometry. World Journal of Surgery. 2008;**32**:2668-2674. DOI: 10.1007/s00268-008-9752-0

[53] Makuuchi M, Kosuge T, Takayama T, Yamazaki S, Kakazu T, et al. Surgery for small liver cancers. Seminars in Surgical Oncology. 1993;**9**:298-304. DOI: 10.1002/ssu.2980090404

[54] Lam CM, Fan ST, Lo CM, Wong J. Major hepatectomy for hepatocellular carcinoma in patients with an unsatisfactory indocyanine green clearance test. The British Journal of Surgery. 1999;**86**:1012-1017. DOI: 10.1046/j.1365-2168.1999.01204.x

[55] Belli G, Fantini C, Belli A, Limongelli P. Laparoscopic liver resection for hepatocellular carcinoma in cirrhosis: Long-term outcomes. Digestive Surgery. 2011;**28**:134-140. DOI: 10.1159/000323824

[56] Paul A, Kaiser GM, Molmenti EP, Schroeder T, Vernadakis S, et al. Klatskin tumors and the accuracy of the bismuth-corlette classification. The American Surgeon. 2011;**77**:1695-1699

[57] Park J, Kim MH, Kim KP, Park DH, Moon SH, et al. Natural history and prognostic factors of advanced

cholangiocarcinoma without surgery, chemotherapy, or radiotherapy: A large-scale observational study. Gut Liver. 2009;**3**:298-305. DOI: 10.5009/gnl.2009.3.4.298

[58] Zervos EE, Osborne D, Goldin SB, Villadolid DV, Thometz DP, et al. Stage does not predict survival after resection of hilar cholangiocarcinomas promoting an aggressive operative approach. American Journal of Surgery. 2005;**190**:810-815. DOI: 10.1016/j.amjsurg.2005.07.025

[59] Jarnagin W, Winston C. Hilar cholangiocarcinoma: Diagnosis and staging. HPB. 2005;7:244-251. DOI: 10.1080/13651820500372533

[60] Soares K, Kamel I, Cosgrove D, Herman J, Pawlik T. Hilar cholangiocarcinoma: Diagnosis, treatment options, and management. Hepatobiliary Surgery and Nutrition. 2014;**3**:18-34. DOI: 10.3978/j.issn.2304-3881.2014.02.05

[61] Deoliveira ML, Schulick RD, Nimura Y, Rosen C, Gores G, et al. New staging system and a registry for perihilar cholangiocarcinoma. Hepatology. 2011;**53**:1363-1371. DOI: 10.1002/hep.24227

[62] Shimada K, Sano T, Sakamoto Y, Esaki M, Kosuge T, et al. Surgical outcomes of the mass-forming plus periductal infiltrating types of intrahepatic cholangiocarcinoma: A comparative study with the typical mass-forming type of intrahepatic cholangiocarcinoma. World Journal of Surgery. 2007;**31**:2016-2022. DOI: 10.1007/s00268-007-9194-0

[63] Sakamoto E, Nimura Y, Hayakawa N, Kamiya J, Kondo S, et al. The pattern of infiltration at the proximal border of hilar bile duct carcinoma: A histologic analysis of 62 resected cases. Annals of Surgery. 1998;**227**:405-411. DOI: 10.1097/00000658-199803000-00013

[64] Hong SM, Pawlik TM, Cho HJ, Aggarwal B, Goggins M, et al. Depth of tumor invasion better predicts prognosis than the current american joint committee on cancer T classification for distal bile duct carcinoma. Surgery. 2009;**146**:250-257. DOI: 10.1016/j.surg.2009.02.023

[65] Murakami Y, Uemura K, Hayashidani Y, Sudo T, Hashimoto Y, et al. Prognostic significance of lymph node metastasis and surgical margin status for distal cholangiocarcinoma. Journal of Surgical Oncology. 2007;**95**:207-212. DOI: 10.1002/jso.20668

[66] Yoshida T, Matsumoto T, Sasaki A, Morii Y, Shibata K, et al. Lymphatic spread differs according to tumor location in extrahepatic bile duct cancer. Hepato-Gastroenterology. 2003;**50**:17-20

Section 3

Gallbladder Carcinoma

Chapter 4

Surgical Advances in the Treatment of Gallbladder Carcinoma at Different Stages

Nicolae Bacalbasa, Irina Balescu, Simona Dima and Irinel Popescu

Abstract

Gallbladder carcinoma remains the most common cancer originating from the biliary tract, which is associated with poor prognosis and poor survival rates. It is estimated that only one-third of patients with histopathological diagnostic of gallbladder cancer had been correctly diagnosed preoperatively, in the remaining cases the diagnostic being established intraoperatively or postoperatively, based on the histopathological examination. Moreover, although surgery remains the most appropriate therapeutic approach in order to improve survival, it is estimated that only 25% of cases with gallbladder carcinomas present resectable lesions. The current chapter reviews the most appropriate surgical options in patients diagnosed with both early stage and advanced stage gallbladder cancer, by minimally invasive as well as by open approach. In the meantime, the therapeutic strategies in incidentally diagnosed gallbladder cancer will be discussed.

Keywords: gallbladder cancer, atypical hepatic resection, bile duct resection, lymph node dissection, survival

1. Introduction

Gallbladder carcinoma represents the most frequently encountered malignant tumor originating from the biliary tract, with a low rate of diagnostic, a low rate of surgical treatment, and an extremely poor long-term prognostic [1, 2].

The global incidence of gallbladder cancer is low (<2/100,000 cases), but significant differences given by the regional and racial criteria have been reported [3].

Therefore, it has been demonstrated that women are more commonly affected by this malignancy; in regard to the patients' age, it seems that the incidence of gallbladder cancer significantly increases after the age of 40. In terms of race, it seems that the highest risk for gallbladder carcinoma has been reported among people from Chile, Poland, India, Japan, and Israel [4].

As for the risk factors incriminated for gallbladder cancer development, it seems that the presence and the dimensions of gallstones increased the body mass index as well as multiparity significantly influence it [5, 6].

2. Treatment options in gallbladder carcinoma

Surgery remains the most efficient therapeutic strategy in order to achieve long-term survival in gallbladder carcinoma patients. However, only a limited number of cases diagnosed with this pathology are amenable to surgery due to the extent of the disease. A generic observation pointed out that only one-third of gallbladder cancer patients are diagnosed preoperatively, and, among these cases, only one quart present resectable lesions [7, 8].

Incidental gallbladder carcinoma also represents a rare condition, ranging from less than 3% of all cases; however, it seems that that this situation is more common in female patients, over 65 years of age who are known with gallbladder stones or cholecystitis and originating from Asian or African descendants [9–11]. In order to provide a rapid diagnostic in such cases, intraoperative frozen section examinations have been proposed with good results [12]. As for the diagnostic criteria of incidental gallbladder carcinoma, certain authors proposed that in this category cases in which the diagnostic is not suspected during surgery or on gross examination of the specimen should be included, the neoplastic process being only detected at the histopathological examination [13].

When it comes to the extent of the resection, this parameter is dictated by the stage of the tumor; however, improvement of the surgical techniques in regard to liver resection and even liver transplantation as well as in regard to the perioperative management of these patients conducted to an increasing number of cases who can benefit from radical surgery for gallbladder carcinoma [14, 15]. Cases presenting advanced stage disease which is no longer amenable to surgery with curative intent can also benefit from palliative procedures in order to minimize the effects of gastrointestinal or biliary obstruction [2]. In selected cases adjuvant therapies such as chemotherapy or radiotherapy might be also associated in order to improve the overall outcomes [2].

3. Surgery as a therapeutic option in gallbladder carcinoma patients

The aggressivity of gallbladder cancer was maybe best defined by Alfred Blalock, an American surgeon who stated in 1924 that "in malignancy of the gallbladder, when a diagnosis can be made without exploration, no operation should be performed, inasmuch as it only shortens the patient's life" [7]. This statement was unfortunately confirmed by a latter publication which demonstrated that on a group of 6222 patients, the cumulative survival rate was of 5–8 months, while the 5-year survival rate did not surpass 4% [16].

However, in the next decades, due to the improvement of the surgical techniques, more extended resections have been safely performed in order to cure this malignancy. This fact was maybe best demonstrated by a Canadian study which analyzed the outcomes of patients submitted to surgery for gallbladder cancer during a 12-year period; cases submitted to surgery in the second part of this interval reported an overall 5-year survival rate of 35%, significantly higher than the first period (in which the 5-year overall survival rate did not surpass 7%) [17].

Whenever gallbladder cancer is suspected, the therapeutic desiderate consists of complete tumoral resection with negative resection margins. In early stages of the disease, this desiderate is achieved if cholecystectomy en bloc with the surrounding liver bed and the regional lymph nodes are excised. In cases in which surgery is planned for a presumed benign disease and at the time of exploration the suspicion of malignancy is raised, hepatic resection should be associated; however, if the surgical team is not prepared to perform liver resection, the patient should be transferred in a specialized center in order to be submitted to a complete surgical procedure. This sequencing of the surgical procedure seems not to influence the long-term survival of the patient [7, 18].

In cases diagnosed in early stages of the disease, it seems that a simple cholecystectomy is enough in order to achieve a good control of the disease; therefore, in stage T1a tumors, the rate of cure after simple cholecystectomy ranges between 85 and 100% [19, 20], while in stage T1b tumors, a more extended local resection should be performed in order to control the disease [21]. This extended resection usually refers to the necessity of associating a wedge hepatic resection [22].

Whenever a T2 gallbladder carcinoma is suspected, a more aggressive surgical procedure including adjacent liver resection involving the segments IVb and V and regional lymph node dissection should be added to improve the outcomes; therefore, it is estimated that, while in cases diagnosed with stage T2 gallbladder cancer, the 5-year overall survival reaches 80% if an extended surgical procedure is performed, significantly higher than simple cholecystectomy (in these cases, the 5-year overall survival ranges between 20 and 40%) [23, 24]. The necessity of resecting segments IVb/Vb is explained by the venous drainage of the gallbladder, which seems to be directed in this area [25].

An interesting study regarding the most appropriate surgical strategy in cases suspected for early gallbladder carcinoma diagnosed during or after cholecystectomy was conducted by Nitta et al. and was published in the Annals of Medicine and Surgery in 2018 [12]; the study included 529 patients submitted to cholecystectomy in Medico Shunju Shiroyama Hospital, Osaka, Japan, between April 2009 and December 2017. Among these cases, there were eight cases diagnosed with gallbladder cancer; five out of the eight cases were submitted to surgery for stones, while the remaining three cases were submitted to surgery for cholecystitis.

Whenever gallbladder cancer was proven at the frozen section, conversion to open surgery occurred, and the patient was submitted to gallbladder bed resection, liver resection of the segments IVb–Vb alone or in association with lymph node dissection; in the meantime if invasion of the cystic duct stump was found, prophylactic common bile duct excision was associated. After a median follow-up period of 17.9 months, five out of the eight patients were still alive; one patient initially diagnosed with stage IIIA gallbladder cancer died due to peritoneal carcinomatosis, while the other two cases died from other diseases [12].

Another interesting topic when it comes to incidental gallbladder carcinoma regards the timing of reoperation; therefore, if the patient is submitted to surgery for presumed benign pathology of the gallbladder and the histopathological studies demonstrate the presence of a malignant transformation at this level, it seems that the best outcomes are reported if early reoperation is performed. Therefore, in the study conducted by Muratore et al. on 11 patients with incidental gallbladder cancer, the authors demonstrated that the best long-term outcomes were seen if radical resection was performed within the first 2.2 months after cholecystectomy [26].

Moreover, the extent of the liver resection should be established in concordance with the local aspect: if the right portal pedicle seems to be involved, liver resection should consist of a right hepatectomy.

In cases suitable for both wedge resection and typical hepatectomy, the extent of liver resection should be carefully tailored due to the fact that in certain cases wedge resection might be insufficient (and associated with positive resection margins), while typical resection might be associated with increased morbidity rates; moreover, the decision of performing a right hepatectomy in patients associating cirrhosis should be taken after analyzing the risk of an insufficient liver remnant [25].

Study, year	No of cases	Stage at surgery	Type of surgery	Recurrence rate	Sites of recurrence	Lymph node metastasis rate	Survival rate	Gallbladder carcinoma related death	Factors influencing survival
Lee (review study) [32]	1266	T1a—706 cases T1b—560 cases	Laparoscopic cholecystectomy	1.1%	Common bile duct	2.5% (10.9% of T1b lesions and 1.8% of T1a lesions)	100% at 5-year follow-up	Eight cases with T1a lesions and 52 cases with T1b lesions died due to recurrent disease	
Nitta (single-center study) [12]	8	Tis—2 cases T1b—1 pt. T2—3 cases	Laparoscopic cholecystectomy—5 cases Open cholecystectomy—3 cases Wedge resection of the gallbladder bed—2 cases Segmental resection—1 case	12.5%	Peritoneal	NR	After a median follow-up period of 17.9 months, one case died due to the progression of the disease, while other two cases died due to other causes	One case— peritoneal carcinomatosis	
Aldossary (single-center study) [33]	76	Stage I—3 cases Stage IIA—13 cases Stage IIB—1 pt. Stage IIIB—2 cases Stage IVB—57 cases	21 cases—resection 55 cases—unresectable lesions	10.5%	NR	NR	20.5% for the entire cohort	71% of cases presented with unresectable lesions and died of disease	Resectability of the lesions Stage at diagnostic

Study, year	No of cases	Stage at surgery	Type of surgery	Recurrence rate	Sites of recurrence	Lymph node metastasis rate	Survival rate	Gallbladder carcinoma related death	Factors influencing survival
Shen (multicentric study) [2]	2379	Stage I—3.6% Stage II—7.3% Stage III A—341 cases Stage IIIB—333 cases Stage IVA—253 cases Stage IVB—838 cases NR—108 cases	Radical resection—641 cases Extended radical resection—82 cases Palliative surgery—499 cases Drainage—261 cases	NR	NR	29.7%	NR	NR	NR
Yildirim (single-center study) [34]	65	T1a—5 cases T1b—8 cases T2—34 cases T3—18 cases	Extended cholecystectomy—28 cases Simple cholecystectomy—37 cases	83.00%	NR	NR	Median survival—41 months 5-year overall survival rate—32%	45 cases	Lymph node status Tumor stage Type of surgery Vascular/neural invasion

Study, year	No of cases	Stage at surgery	Type of surgery	Recurrence rate	Sites of recurrence	Lymph node metastasis rate	Survival rate	Gallbladder carcinoma related death	Factors influencing survival
Jin (multicentric study) [35]	613	NR	Cholecystectomy—150 cases Partial hepatectomy—249 cases Extensive hepatectomy—25 cases Palliative/other procedures—108 cases Diagnostic—81 cases	NR	NR	NR	NR	NR	NR
Creasy, single-center study [36]	74	IIIA—2 cases IIIB—10 cases IVA—6 cases IVB—43 cases	Surgery with curative intent including resection of segments 4 and 5—6 cases Hemihepatectomy—2 cases Extended hepatectomy—2 cases Bile duct resection—10 cases	NR	NR	NR	Median overall survival—14.2 months	61 cases died due to the progression of the disease	Completeness of cytoreduction

Table 1.
The largest studies conducted on the theme of the role of surgical approach in gallbladder cancer patients.

Whenever extended liver resections are expected with a future liver remnant lesser than 25%, a portal vein embolization might be taken into consideration [27]. Another interesting subject is the one regarding the necessity of routinely association of caudate lobe resection; while the Japanese surgeons stand for routine caudate lobe resection, in the Western countries this practice is not part of the standard protocol [25, 28].

When it comes to the lymphatic spread of gallbladder cancer, anatomy studies demonstrated that the first involved lymph nodes are located along the biliary tree and represented by the cystic, common hepatic, and common bile duct lymph nodes; going further, the next involved stations are located along the pancreaticoduodenal, common hepatic artery, and coeliac axis nodes. The most distant lymph node stations are located at the level of the pancreatic body and tail; whenever tumoral cells are encountered at this level, the case is considered to have distant metastases [29].

As for the extent of the lymph node dissection, different opinions have been proposed so far: since certain authors recommended a local lymph node dissection involving the stations from the hepatoduodenal ligament, other surgeons routinely associate retropancreatic and celiac trunk lymph node dissection [7].

In cases presenting more advanced stages of the disease such as T3 gallbladder carcinomas, more extended upper abdominal resections might be taken into consideration; if the tumoral process involves the biliary duct, bile duct resection and anastomosis should be performed. Moreover if the adjacent organs (such as gastrointestinal tract or colon) are involved, segmental resections might be needed in order to achieve complete resection of the malignant process.

Special care should be provided for cases associating gallbladder cancer and stones; such patients might present local adhesions which might induce a difficult differentiation between the inflammatory and malignant transformations; therefore, a large resection is advisable in order to avoid incomplete resection. Whenever the desiderate of negative resection margins is achieved, long-term survival should be expected; in such cases the rate of 5-year overall survival ranges between 30 and 50% [30, 31].

Contrarily, patients diagnosed with stage T4 gallbladder lesions report a poor outcome, surgery with curative intent being suitable in rare cases. In such patients surgery is most commonly performed with palliative intent, while the overall survival remains extremely poor.

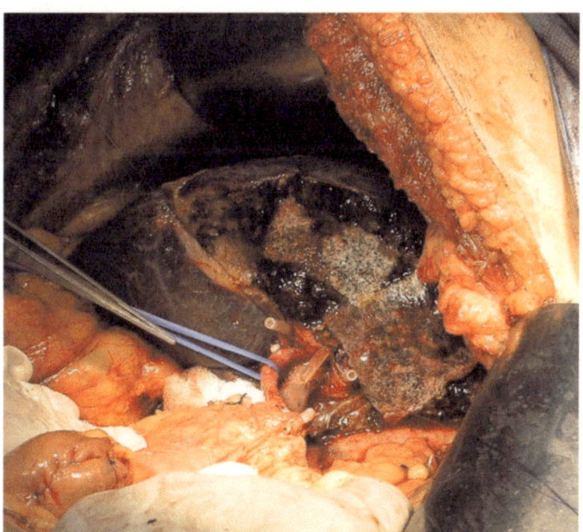

Figure 1.
Intraoperative aspect after right hepatectomy extended to the caudate lobe for locally advanced gallbladder carcinoma. Association of common bile duct resection was performed.

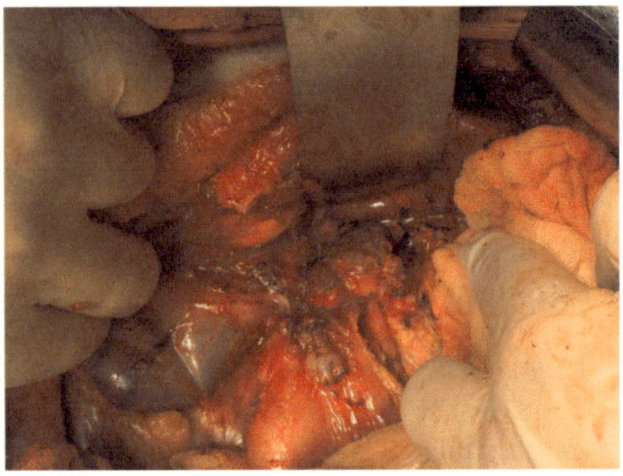

Figure 2.
Incidental finding—gallbladder carcinoma.

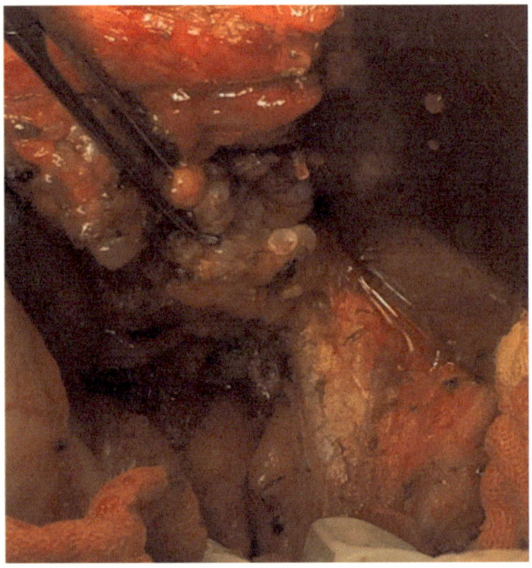

Figure 3.
Dissection of the cystic duct.

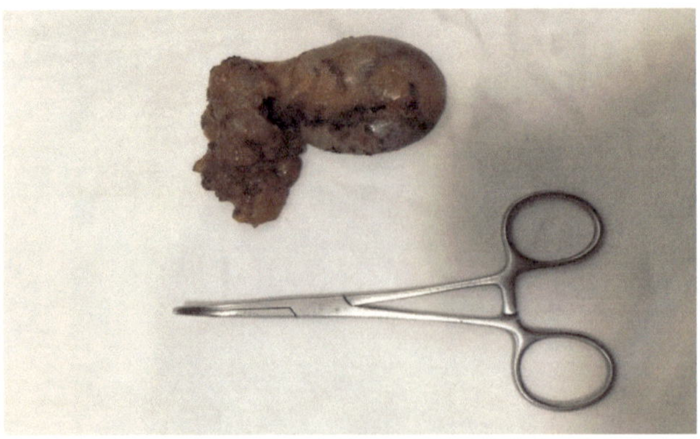

Figure 4.
The final aspect after cholecystectomy en bloc with lymph node excision.

The largest studies, which were focused on the role of surgery in gallbladder cancer patients, are summarized in **Table 1**.

Intraoperative aspects of patients submitted to surgery for gallbladder carcinoma are shown in **Figures 1–4**.

4. Laparoscopic versus open approach in gallbladder cancer patients

Although laparoscopic cholecystectomy represents one of the most facile to be performed minimally invasive procedures, there is still controversy regarding the feasibility and safety of the laparoscopic approach in gallbladder cancer patients. This fact is explained through the aspect that in such cases multiple upper abdominal resections might be needed in order to control the disease; moreover, another fact that should be taken into consideration when deciding for a minimally invasive approach in gallbladder patients is related to the risk of port-site metastases development.

One of the most recent studies which envisaged the efficacy and safety of the laparoscopic approach in gallbladder cancer patients has been recently published by the Chinese surgeons from Jiangsu [37]. The authors included in their study 102 patients with gallbladder carcinoma who were submitted to surgery between August 2008 and August 2017 in a minimally invasive manner, 41 cases, or via an open approach, 61 cases.

The authors demonstrated that there was no significant difference between the operative blood loss, operative time, postoperative complications, R0 resection, and tumor-related death between the two groups [37]. Moreover, the authors demonstrated an improved postoperative outcome for patients submitted to a minimally invasive procedure, while the long-term outcomes demonstrated similar overall survival rates at 1 year, 3 years, and 5 years postoperatively. Moreover, the authors analyzed the 5-year survival rate according to the stage at the initial diagnostic and demonstrated that there was no significant difference in terms of survival for patients submitted to surgery for Tis, T1b, T2, and T3 tumors in a minimally invasive or open approach.

In terms of recurrences and metastases, the authors reported that there was no difference in regard to the incisional site metastases between the two groups (4.9% in the laparoscopic group and 3.3% in the open approach group). However, the authors demonstrated that the risk of incisional metastases was increased in cases presenting gallbladder rupture.

When it came to the recurrence time, it seems that patients submitted to an open approach experienced relapsed disease earlier than those submitted to a minimally invasive approach; however, this aspect was rather related to the fact that among patients submitted to an open approach, a higher proportion of T3 tumors existed [37].

The subject of port-site metastases has been widely studied so far, in certain cases excision of the port sites being proposed in order to minimize this risk [38, 39].

One of the largest studies which debated the role of port-site resection in laparoscopically treated gallbladder cancer patients was conducted by Fuks et al. and was published in the Journal of Visceral Surgery [40]. The study included 218 patients with incidental gallbladder cancer who had been treated in a minimally invasive manner between 1998 and 2008 in 21 centers in France; among these cases, re-resection with curative intent was performed in 148 cases, 54 cases being also submitted to port-site excision.

Their results were compared to the ones reported in the remaining 94 patients who did not undergo to port-site excision. There was no significant difference between the two groups in terms of tumor stage or extent of resection. Port-site metastases were encountered in a single patient who had been previously submitted to port-site excision; it was the case of a patient who had been initially submitted to surgery for a T3 gallbladder carcinoma and who died 15 months after resection due to the development of peritoneal carcinomatosis.

However, the authors demonstrated that the 1-year, 3-year, and 5-year overall survival rates were similar between the two categories of patients; moreover, patients submitted to port-site excision developed an incisional hernia rate at the site of port excision of 8% [40].

Therefore, the authors concluded that port-site excision should not be routinely performed in such cases; an interesting aspect that was pointed out by the same study was the one regarding the possible protective role, which could be given by peritoneal frozen section surrounding the peritoneal trocar orifices in cases presenting greater or equal to T2 tumors [40].

5. Postoperative complications after surgery for gallbladder carcinoma

Whenever surgery with curative intent is performed in gallbladder carcinoma patients, the postoperative risk of developing complications seems to remain high at both 30 and 90 days postoperatively. Therefore, although most studies take into consideration the 30-day morbidity/mortality rate, it seems that maybe a more adequate tool in order to quantify the postoperative outcomes is represented by the 90-day morbidity/mortality rate. This fact seems to be true not only in gallbladder cancer patients but also in other malignancies such as pancreatic cancer and esophageal or gastric cancer [41, 42].

A recent study conducted on this theme by Goussous et al. and published in 2017 demonstrated that the postoperative mortality within the first 90 days postoperatively is 2.3-fold higher than the 30-day postoperative mortality [43]. Another interesting aspect underlined by this study was the one that the 30-day and 90-day mortality, respectively, was significantly correlated with the degree of tumoral differentiation, with the presence of vascular and lymphatic invasion, with the stage of the tumor, with incomplete resection, and with low-volume centers. Moreover, the authors demonstrated the fact that even in cases submitted to surgery in a minimally invasive manner, the 90-day mortality rate was significantly higher than the 30-day mortality rate [43].

6. Factors predicting survival after surgery for gallbladder cancer

It seems that the most important prognostic factors predicting the long-term outcomes after surgery for gallbladder carcinoma remain the stage of the disease at the time of diagnostic (including tumoral and lymph node status) as well as the completeness of resection [7, 18]. In the meantime, association of clinical signs as jaundice is most often a sign of locally advanced/unresectable disease and therefore is associated with poor rates of survival [44].

One of the most recent studies which were conducted on the theme of predictors of curative resection and long-term survival in patients with gallbladder cancer was published by Mishra et al. in the American Journal of Surgery [45]. The study included 385 patients diagnosed with gallbladder cancer between September 2003 and December 2014 in the Academic Block, GB Pant Hospital, New Delhi, India.

The authors demonstrated that cases presenting gastric outlet obstruction, weight loss, abdominal lump, and obstructive jaundice were more likely to present unresectable lesions.

Moreover, patients presenting at the time of initial diagnostic obstructive jaundice presented significantly lower rates of 1-year, 3-year and 5-year overall survival than those in whom jaundice had not been present at the time of diagnostic [45].

7. Palliative surgery for unresectable/metastatic gallbladder cancer

Due to the fact that a large proportion of patients with gallbladder cancer are diagnosed in advanced stages of the disease, when surgery with curative intent is no longer possible, palliative procedures might be needed in order to alleviate the symptoms. In such cases, the most frequently reported symptoms necessitating palliative procedures are represented by pruritus, cholangitis, jaundice, digestive obstruction, or pain. However, in this subgroup of patients, the goal of surgery is a pure palliative one, the overall survival ranging between 2 and 4 months [46, 47].

8. Conclusions

Gallbladder carcinoma remains an extremely aggressive malignancy which is rarely diagnosed in early stages of the disease; therefore the overall survival rates remain extremely poor, the most important predictors for long-term survival being related to the stage at diagnostic as well as to the completeness of resection. However, it should not be omitted the fact that most often extended upper abdominal resections might be needed in order to achieve an R0 resection; therefore such patients should be addressed in high-volume centers.

Acknowledgements

This work was supported by the project number PN-III-P1-1.2-PCCDI-2017-0797 and project title “Pathogenic mechanisms and personalized treatment in pancreatic cancer using multi-omics technologies.”

Author details

Nicolae Bacalbasa[1,2*], Irina Balescu[3], Simona Dima[2,4] and Irinel Popescu[4,5]

1 "Carol Davila" University of Medicine and Pharmacy, Bucharest, Romania

2 Center of Excellence in Translational Medicine, Fundeni Clinical Institute, Bucharest, Romania

3 Ponderas Academic Hospital, Bucharest, Romania

4 "Dan Setlacec" Center of Gastrointestinal Disease and Liver Transplantation, Fundeni Clinical Institute, Bucharest, Romania

5 "Titu Maiorescu" University, Bucharest, Romania

*Address all correspondence to: nicolae_bacalbasa@yahoo.ro

References

[1] Wistuba II, Gazdar AF. Gallbladder cancer: Lessons from a rare tumour. Nature Reviews. Cancer. 2004;**4**(9): 695-706

[2] Shen HX, Song HW, Xu XJ, Jiao ZY, Ti ZY, Li ZY, et al. Clinical epidemiological survey of gallbladder carcinoma in northwestern China, 2009-2013: 2379 cases in 17 centers. Chronic Diseases and Translational Medicine. 2017;**3**(1):60-66

[3] Hundal R, Shaffer EA. Gallbladder cancer: Epidemiology and outcome. Clinical Epidemiology. 2014;**6**:99-109

[4] Randi G, Franceschi S, La Vecchia C. Gallbladder cancer worldwide: Geographical distribution and risk factors. International Journal of Cancer. 2006;**118**(7):1591-1602

[5] Serra I, Calvo A, Baez S, Yamamoto M, Endoh K, Aranda W. Risk factors for gallbladder cancer. An international collaborative case-control study. Cancer. 1996;**78**(7):1515-1517

[6] Engeland A, Tretli S, Austad G, Bjorge T. Height and body mass index in relation to colorectal and gallbladder cancer in two million Norwegian men and women. Cancer Causes & Control. 2005;**16**(8):987-996

[7] Miller G, Jarnagin WR. Gallbladder carcinoma. European Journal of Surgical Oncology. 2008;**34**(3):306-312

[8] Goetze T, Paolucci V. Does laparoscopy worsen the prognosis for incidental gallbladder cancer? Surgical Endoscopy. 2006;**20**(2):286-293

[9] Sikora SS, Singh RK. Surgical strategies in patients with gallbladder cancer: Nihilism to optimism. Journal of Surgical Oncology. 2006;**93**(8):670-681

[10] Chan SY, Poon RT, Lo CM, Ng KK, Fan ST. Management of carcinoma of the gallbladder: A single-institution experience in 16 years. Journal of Surgical Oncology. 2008;**97**(2): 156-164

[11] Yamamoto H, Hayakawa N, Kitagawa Y, Katohno Y, Sasaya T, Takara D, et al. Unsuspected gallbladder carcinoma after laparoscopic cholecystectomy. Journal of Hepato-Biliary-Pancreatic Surgery. 2005;**12**(5): 391-398

[12] Nitta T, Kataoka J, Ohta M, Fujii K, Takashima Y, Inoue Y, et al. Surgical strategy for suspected early gallbladder carcinoma including incidental gallbladder carcinoma diagnosed during or after cholecystectomy. Annals of Medicine and Surgery (London). 2018;**33**:56-59

[13] Behari A, Kapoor VK. Incidental gall bladder cancer. Advances in Surgery. 2013;**47**:227-249

[14] Nishio H, Nagino M, Ebata T, Yokoyama Y, Igami T, Nimura Y. Aggressive surgery for stage IV gallbladder carcinoma; What are the contraindications? Journal of Hepato-Biliary-Pancreatic Surgery. 2007;**14**(4): 351-357

[15] Hemming AW, Magliocca JF, Fujita S, Kayler LK, Hochwald S, Zendejas I, et al. Combined resection of the liver and pancreas for malignancy. Journal of the American College of Surgeons. 2010; **210**(5):808-806

[16] Piehler JM, Crichlow RW. Primary carcinoma of the gallbladder. Surgery, Gynecology & Obstetrics. 1978;**147**(6): 929-942

[17] Dixon E, Vollmer CM Jr, Sahajpal A, Cattral M, Grant D, Doig C, et al. An

aggressive surgical approach leads to improved survival in patients with gallbladder cancer: A 12-year study at a North American Center. Annals of Surgery. 2005;**241**(3):385-394

[18] Fong Y, Jarnagin W, Blumgart LH. Gallbladder cancer: Comparison of patients presenting initially for definitive operation with those presenting after prior noncurative intervention. Annals of Surgery. 2000; **232**(4):557-569

[19] Yamaguchi K, Tsuneyoshi M. Subclinical gallbladder carcinoma. American Journal of Surgery. 1992; **163**(4):382-386

[20] Shirai Y, Yoshida K, Tsukada K, Muto T. In apparent carcinoma of the gallbladder. An appraisal of a radical second operation after simple cholecystectomy. Annals of Surgery. 1992;**215**(4):326-331

[21] Principe A, Del Gaudio M, Ercolani G, Golfieri R, Cucchetti A, Pinna AD. Radical surgery for gallbladder carcinoma: Possibilities of survival. Hepato-Gastroenterology. 2006;**53**(71): 660-664

[22] Tsuji T, Kanemitsu K, Hiraoka T, Takamori H, Toyama E, Tanaka H, et al. A new method to establish the rational extent of hepatic resection for advanced gallbladder cancer using dye injection through the cystic artery. HPB: The Official Journal of the International Hepato Pancreato Biliary Association. 2004;**6**(1):33-66

[23] de Aretxabala XA, Roa IS, Burgos LA, Araya JC, Villaseca MA, Silva JA. Curative resection in potentially resectable tumours of the gallbladder. The European Journal of Surgery. 1997; **163**(6):419-426

[24] Oertli D, Herzog U, Tondelli P. Primary carcinoma of the gallbladder: Operative experience during a 16 year period. The European Journal of Surgery. 1993;**159**(8):415-420

[25] Pilgrim CH, Usatoff V, Evans P. Consideration of anatomical structures relevant to the surgical strategy for managing gallbladder carcinoma. European Journal of Surgical Oncology. 2009;**35**(11):1131-1136

[26] Muratore A, Amisano M, Vigano L, Massucco P, Capussotti L. Gallbladder cancer invading the perimuscular connective tissue: Results of reresection after prior non-curative operation. Journal of Surgical Oncology. 2003; **83**(4):212-215

[27] Reddy SK, Marroquin CE, Kuo PC, Pappas TN, Clary BM. Extended hepatic resection for gallbladder cancer. American Journal of Surgery. 2007; **194**(3):355-361

[28] Reid KM, Ramos-De la Medina A, Donohue JH. Diagnosis and surgical management of gallbladder cancer: A review. Journal of Gastrointestinal Surgery. 2007;**11**(5):671-681

[29] Mekeel KL, Hemming AW. Surgical management of gallbladder carcinoma: A review. Journal of Gastrointestinal Surgery. 2007;**11**(9):1188-1193

[30] Chijiiwa K, Tanaka M. Carcinoma of the gallbladder: An appraisal of surgical resection. Surgery. 1994;**115**(6): 751-756

[31] Bartlett DL, Fong Y, Fortner JG, Brennan MF, Blumgart LH. Long-term results after resection for gallbladder cancer. Implications for staging and management. Annals of Surgery. 1996; **224**(5):639-646

[32] Lee SE, Jang JY, Lim CS, Kang MJ, Kim SW. Systematic review on the surgical treatment for T1 gallbladder cancer. World Journal of Gastroentero-logy. 2011;**17**(2):174-180

[33] Aldossary MY, Alayed AA, Amr SS, Alqahtani S, Alnahawi M, Alqahtani MS. Gallbladder cancer in Eastern Province of Saudi Arabia: A retrospective cohort study. Annals of Medicine and Surgery (London). 2018;**35**:117-123

[34] Yildirim E, Celen O, Gulben K, Berberoglu U. The surgical management of incidental gallbladder carcinoma. European Journal of Surgical Oncology. 2005;**31**(1):45-52

[35] Jin LX, Pitt SC, Hall BL, Pitt HA. Aggressive surgical management of gallbladder cancer: At what cost? Surgery. 2013;**154**(2):266-273

[36] Creasy JM, Goldman DA, Dudeja V, Lowery MA, Cercek A, Balachandran VP, et al. Systemic chemotherapy combined with resection for locally advanced gallbladder carcinoma: Surgical and survival outcomes. Journal of the American College of Surgeons. 2017;**224**(5):906-916

[37] Feng JW, Yang XH, Liu CW, Wu BQ, Sun DL, Chen XM, et al. Comparison of laparoscopic and open approach in treating gallbladder cancer. The Journal of Surgical Research. 2019; **234**:269-276

[38] Hu JB, Sun XN, Xu J, He C. Port site and distant metastases of gallbladder cancer after laparoscopic cholecystectomy diagnosed by positron emission tomography. World Journal of Gastroenterology. 2008;**14**(41): 6428-6431

[39] Giuliante F, Ardito F, Vellone M, Clemente G, Nuzzo G. Port-sites excision for gallbladder cancer incidentally found after laparoscopic cholecystectomy. American Journal of Surgery. 2006;**191**(1):114-116

[40] Fuks D, Regimbeau JM, Pessaux P, Bachellier P, Raventos A, Mantion G, et al. Is port-site resection necessary in the surgical management of gallbladder cancer? Journal of Visceral Surgery. 2013;**150**(4):277-284

[41] Fischer C, Lingsma H, Hardwick R, Cromwell DA, Steyerberg E, Groene O. Risk adjustment models for short-term outcomes after surgical resection for oesophagogastric cancer. The British Journal of Surgery. 2016;**103**(1):105-116

[42] Swanson RS, Pezzi CM, Mallin K, Loomis AM, Winchester DP. The 90-day mortality after pancreatectomy for cancer is double the 30-day mortality: More than 20,000 resections from the national cancer data base. Annals of Surgical Oncology. 2014;**21**(13): 4059-4067

[43] Goussous N, Hosseini M, Sill AM, Cunningham SC. Minimally invasive and open gallbladder cancer resections: 30- vs 90-day mortality. Hepatobiliary & Pancreatic Diseases International. 2017;**16**(4):405-411

[44] Hawkins WG, DeMatteo RP, Jarnagin WR, Ben Porat L, Blumgart LH, Fong Y. Jaundice predicts advanced disease and early mortality in patients with gallbladder cancer. Annals of Surgical Oncology. 2004;**11**(3):310-315

[45] Mishra PK, Saluja SS, Prithiviraj N, Varshney V, Goel N, Patil N. Predictors of curative resection and long term survival of gallbladder cancer–A retrospective analysis. American Journal of Surgery. 2017;**214**(2):278-286

[46] Kapoor VK, Pradeep R, Haribhakti SP, Singh V, Sikora SS, Saxena R, et al. Intrahepatic segment III cholangiojejunostomy in advanced carcinoma of the gallbladder. The British Journal of Surgery. 1996;**83**(12):1709-1711

[47] Miller G, Boman J, Shrier I, Gordon PH. Small-bowel obstruction secondary to malignant disease: An 11-year audit. Canadian Journal of Surgery. 2000; **43**(5):353-358

Section 4

Peri-Hilar or Hilar Cholangiocarcinoma

Chapter 5

Perihilar or (Hilar) Cholangiocarcinoma: Interventional to Surgical Management

Pankaj Prasoon, Kohei Miura, Kizuki Yuza, Yuki Hirose, Jun Sakata and Toshifumi Wakai

Abstract

Peri-hilar cholangiocarcinoma (PHC) or hilar cholangiocarcinoma (HCCA) characterizes a critical effort to assess significantly sick patients. The existing scenery and proof to the diagnosis and treatments for hilar cholangiocarcinoma are improving day by day. Patients with HCCA encounter numerous obstacles in acquiring efficient therapies. The condition is uncommon, and the majority patients don't have any distinct risk factors, doing selection process inadequate. The initial signs and symptoms in many cases are non-specific, and in many patients the tumors are not resectable because of involvement of the perihilar structures. MRI with MRCP offers further information about the extent of biliary involvement. Furthermore, endoscopic stenting and percutaneous drain could be useful for intricate hilar strictures. Surgical resections with negative margins are related to good likelihood of survival for patients representing with HCCA. Regardless of the accessibility of curative treatment strategies such as operative resection and liver transplantation, most sufferers with HCCA shows with repeated, metastases or locally advanced disease with a poor prognosis. Within this chapter, we have tried to elaborate the modalities of treatment from intervention to surgical approach for HCCA.

Keywords: perihilar cholangiocarcinoma (PHC), hilar cholangiocarcinoma (HCCA), biliary drainage (BD), magnetic resonance cholangiopancreatography (MRCP), surgical resection, magnetic resonance imaging (MRI)

1. Introduction

Perihilar cholangiocarcinoma (PHC) is the typical tumor also referred as Klatskin tumor, is liable for nearly 60% of biliary tract cholangiocarcinoma [1]. These types of tumors develop through the biliary tract epithelium and may even appear in entire intra hepatic biliary duct. It could be subdivided on the basis of their location for instance, intrahepatic, perihilar and distal HCCA [1]. These types of malignancy commence within the extrahepatic bile duct proximal to the origin of the cystic duct. PHC is typically alienated based on Bismuth-Corlette classification in accordance with the proximal magnitude of the tumor into the biliary tract [2].

HCCA incorporates a very poor prognosis, and surgical treatment continues to be the only preventive alternatives. Nevertheless, very few patients are determined in a treatable phase, and palliative remedies are, consequently, necessary. Endoscopy has a beneficial role while in the investigation of the patients with HCCA who definitely are not fit for surgical treatment. Primary sclerosing cholangitis (PSC) is regarded as the prevalent risk factor for PHC in European nations and about 8–40% sufferers acquire this type of malignancy [3]. Hepatobiliary flukes, together with *Clonorchis sinensis* and *Opisthorchis viverrini*, are the risk issues for cholangiocarcinoma in southeast Asian continent [4]. Additional acknowledged risk factors for cholangiocarcinoma are intra-hepatic stones, biliary abnormalities such as Caroli disease, HCV infection, liver cirrhosis and acquaintance to thorium-containing contrast media [5, 6]. Cholangiocarcinoma affects more commonly in men than women, and the Asians are having higher incidence nearly twice over whites and blacks [7].

HCCA frequently reveals an increasingly gradual pattern than intrahepatic cholangiocarcinomas, through which slower tumor progression is ultimately shadowed by permeation of the perihilar region, adenopathy and direct liver invasion. The caudate lobe is generally intricate as a result of additionally direct or ductal invasion [8]. Distant metastasis through the lymphatic system can also take place [9]. The differential diagnosis incorporates benign strictures, including all those attributable to PSC, Mirizzi syndrome, HIV cholangiopathy and postoperative bile duct injuries. Additionally, other tumors, together with lymphoma, can imitate hilar cholangiocarcinoma [9]. The most prevalent clinical manifestation of HCCA is uncomplicated obstructive jaundice. Nevertheless, not all patients having a speculated hilar stricture could have cholangiocarcinoma [10].

Despite the fact that there is dispute in regards to the aftereffect of preoperative biliary decompression on operative consequence in sufferers with malignant biliary blockages, many experts have stated that liver dysfunction attributable to obstructive jaundice might be a considerable risk factor in significant hepatectomy [11–13].

Specifically, when it comes to perihilar cholangiocarcinoma, extended hepatectomy is usually necessary to offer the most effective possibility of treatment. It is actually preferable to conduct preoperative biliary drainage (PBD) for the future remnant liver (FRL) to maintain postoperative liver functionality. Additionally, selective cholangiography by having a PBD catheter generally offers much more specific information regarding the tumor level across the biliary duct [14].

Nevertheless, disputes remain to be around the best way to accomplish PBD in patients with perihilar PHC. There are numerous disagreements within the clinical benefits of percutaneous transhepatic biliary drainage (PTBD) compared to endoscopic biliary drainage (EBD), stated before that may be affected by either (ERBD) endoscopic retrograde biliary drainage or (ENBD) endoscopic nasobiliary drainage. PTBD have been the most favored method for preliminary PBD [15, 16]. Actually, while contemplating PBD it is mandatory to bear in mind about the perils associated with cholangitis, extended pre-operative stay in the hospital, failing to boost the nutritional state and higher post-operative additional complications [17, 18].

2. Preoperative biliary drainage (PBD)

HCCA is usually a tumor of the extrahepatic bile duct relating to the left and right main hepatic duct or their confluence. Biliary drainage in HCCA is oftentimes technically difficult as a consequence of difficulties linked to the degree of biliary obstruction. This could lead to some unfavorable situations, particularly in acute cholangitis. Therefore, the conclusion on the indication and techniques of biliary drainage in patients with HCCA ought to be meticulously assessed [17]. PBD might have additional advantages in selected patients with the extreme lack of nutrition or biliary sepsis as well as in individuals considering the postponed surgical procedure depending upon on (PVE) portal vein embolization or chemo-radio therapy [19]. Furthermore, cholangiography attained by PTBD or ENBD can offer much more specific information relating to the complex segmental anatomy with the intrahepatic bile ducts and also the extent of cancer across the segregated biliary ducts [17].

So far, the ideal serum bilirubin level for surgical treatment has not yet been established. Moreover, the suitable time period of PBD hasn't been evidently established. Extended use of biliary drainage would raise the potential risk of drainage malfunction, tract seeding, and additional inflammatory alterations towards the bile duct.

Even though biliary drainage varies concerning proximal and distal biliary obstructions, most scientific studies reviewed the different degrees of biliary obstruction being a solitary entity [20].

2.1 Percutaneous transhepatic biliary drainage (PTBD)

The potential advantages of preoperative biliary drainage consist of its possible ways to converse with cholestasis-associated hepatic and synthetic ferocity along with improvement of the nutritional status of the body and boosting the immune function [21–23]. The use of multiple catheters along with the contrast agent in PTBD procedure offers drainage of the liver and enables far additional accurate description of the tumor, and could produce added exploratory advantages through surgical observation of the liver hilum [16, 24]. It has been specifically learned that the reintervention rate or even an alternate drainage technique, is commonly reduced PTBD technique when compared to EBD [24, 25]. Kim et al. [22] witnessed a minimal alteration proportion in the PTBD group compared to the EBD group, consistent with other preceding research. Alteration to PTBD within the EBD group was as a result of issues induced by EBD and failure to attain adequate decompression for the FRL. Cholangitis, which is probably the additional complications that may take place following PBD, is really a distinctive dilemma that frequently necessitates reintervention [22]. There could possibly be feasible clarification in EBD group with an increased rate of conversion compared to the PTBD group. Certainly, cholangitis could be the major side-effect of post-ERCP in patients with PHC, as contrast medium is injected into the biliary tract to delineate the tumor that could not subsequently be drained and further it could aggravate the cholangitis.

Regardless of the several advantages of PTBD being a preoperative biliary drainage method, it offers one particular terrific weak point; the potential of cancers dissemination alongside catheter tract. It is really an unalterable event contrary to other additional complications for instance cholangitis, bleeding, and pancreatitis. According to Hwang et al. [26]; 231 patients of PHC gone through PTBD preoperatively revealed that; 4 patients or 1.7% patients encountered recurrence along with the PTBD tract on an average of 13.5 months following surgical procedure. Takahashi et al. [27], described in the patients with PHC and distal cholangiocarcinoma who undergone resection following PTBD, he witnessed recurrence within the PTBD catheter tract in 23 (5.2%) of 445 patients. The authors recommended that likelihood of PTBD tract recurrence could possibly be underrated due to the fact even though metastatic deposits could progress at any site, earlier recognition of recurrence catheter piercing site location for example the skin, abdominal wall, and liver parenchyma, is actually difficult to assess [27]. In the research of

Kim [22] et al., there were 52 patients who went through surgical resection within the PTBD group, two patients (3.8%) got catheter tract site metastasis during the follow-up period. They demonstrated a relatively brief mean time to recurrence as opposed to other 28 patients who encountered tumor recurrence within the PTBD group devoid of catheter tract metastasis (10.5 months vs. 16 months). Preceding researchers have pondered that several catheters drain along with an extended time-span PTBD techniques are probable risk components for catheter tract recurrence [27].

Conferring to Kim et al. [22]; EBD was linked with a higher likelihood of technique associated issues for instance cholangitis and pancreatitis compared to PTBD, understanding that PTBD was linked to a lot fewer complications than EBD, providing a significantly reduced regularity of reintervention following PTBD. On the other hand, these issues were being conveniently handled devoid of intense morbidity in many instances. While the other study outcomes recommend that there might be an edge to utilizing ENBD instead of ERBD for biliary decompression for the FRL. During initial PBD in patients with resectable PHC. PTBD might be of interest the following best alternate when ENBD just isn't attainable or inadequate for biliary decompression as a result of authentic, even though minimal risk of fatal catheter tract metastasis [27].

PTBD allows for accurate lobar selection coupled with lowering the potential risk of unveiling the biliary tree to duodenal contents. This might conceptually enhance the achievement's biliary drainage and prevent cholangitis [28]. Accomplishment of PTBD necessitates slight sedation, hereafter achievable even in unstable or comorbid patients who cannot endure anesthesia [29]. Conversely, PTBD is associated to discomfort and pain to the skin piercing site. Occasionally, PTBD really should be followed up by internalization of stent that might be related to increased infection and bleeding issues [29, 30].

Percutaneous self-expandable metallic stents; could probably be carefully chosen for preparatory biliary drainage in patients with advanced type III or IV hilar cholangiocarcinoma, provided that increased preliminary efficacy and minimal degree of procedure-related cholangitis [31, 32].

Within a recent meta-analysis, it's been demonstrated that PTBD group has considerably greater drainage results when compared with EBD group. Patients who experienced PTBD had comparatively fewer cholangitis attacks; nevertheless, there wasn't any significant difference in pancreatitis and over-all complications within both groups. Fatality rate within 30 days was equivalent within both groups; this might be apt to be as a result of hidden characteristics of the disease by itself. PTBD group, on the other hand, experienced greater post procedure hemorrhage. This may be due to the second step with the PTBD tactic in certain individuals who requires internalization of the stent [33]. Although, PTBD appears allied with substantial postoperative morbidity, additional prospective research is needed in order to determine the suitable method of biliary drainage in PHC [34, 35]. Moreover, PTBD could be challenging as it may cause (PVT) portal vein thrombosis as well it may cause tract related seeding of tumor that could alter operative measures of the tumor [36, 37]. According to latest study [37]; they have stated that PTBD enhances the likelihood of seeding metastasis and reduces the length of the postoperative survival in patients with PHC. Endoscopic biliary drainage is usually recommended because the optimum solution to preoperative biliary drainage [37].

The suitable drainage strategy is still contentious topic, wherein specialists are likely to prefer the percutaneous method with the explanations of straight approachability to bile duct and utilization of the intraluminal drains postoperatively and throughout the hepaticojejunostomy [38].

2.2 Endoscopic retrograde biliary drainage (ERBD) or endoscopic nasobiliary drainage (ENBD)

Furthermore, tumor encasement of portal vessels and bile ducts can result in segmental or lobar atrophy in PHC (**Figure 1**). In patients with PHC, liver resection or lobes can be determined by MDCT (**Figure 2**), and biliary decompression to relieve cholestasis for the FRL [39].

ERBD has some positive aspects of being more physiologic, improves nutrition, decreases endotoxemia, stabilizes lipid alterations, and boosts the immune system capabilities [40]. ENBD is the endorsed approach in several parts of Asia. As with PTBD, it offers much more specific information about the extent of tumor over the biliary ducts [14]. Some authors described fewer difficulties and an extraordinary accomplishment rate of ENBD equated to EBD [25, 41]. Unilateral ENBD into the future remnant lobe(s) demonstrated a higher rate of success, recommending that it must be an efficient and appropriate preoperative drainage means for perihilar cholangiocarcinoma even just in sufferers with B-C type III to IV tumors. At our institute we commonly perform ENBD for pre-operative biliary drainage (**Figure 3**). To scale back the postprocedural issues, ENBD really should be carried out without having EST or pancreatography [41]. The ENBD of HCCA is usually very complicated and sophisticated. ERBD has got the disadvantage of further complicating the intraoperative assessment of the longitudinal tumor expansion and postponing the surgical procedure [24, 42].

Not too long ago, it has been established that ENBD may be the treatment of preference and PTBD could be the second choice. ENBD might be unpleasant, as a result of the nasal catheter, as compared with endoscopic retrograde biliary drainage, utilizing a plastic-type material or expanding metallic stent [41].

Even though we could keep track of real-time bile output in patients with ENBD, earlier recognition of catheter issues regarding the catheter insertion or malfunction with the drainage catheter, for instance blockage or dislocation, is achievable and catheter complication become evident with time-lag offering with segmental cholangitis. Continual jaundice or decline of clinical parameters regarding liver function or systemic inflammation may occur in patients with ERBD [43]. In patients with Bismuth

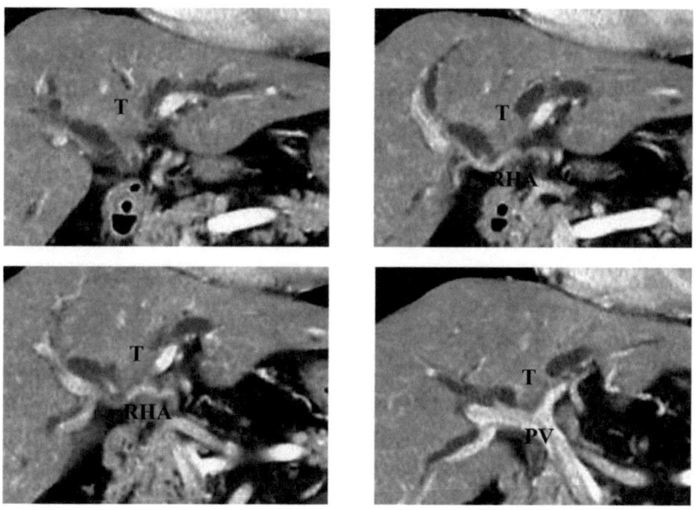

Figure 1.
Abdominal contrast CT examination findings of left sided Bismuth IV type perihilar cholangiocarcinoma. T: tumor, RHA: right hepatic artery, PV: portal vein.

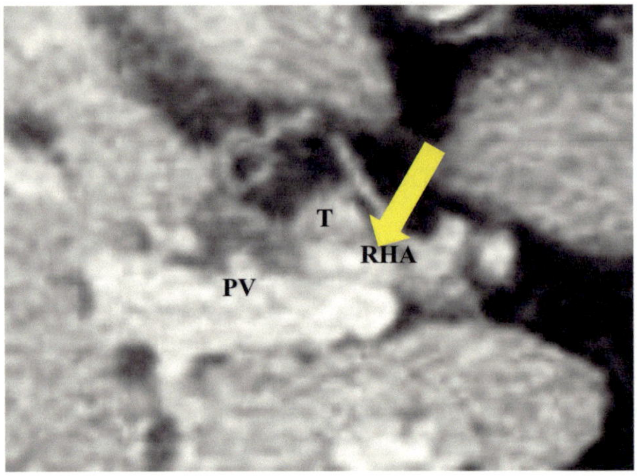

Figure 2.
Abdominal contrast CT showed invasion into the right hepatic artery (yellow arrow) was suspected.

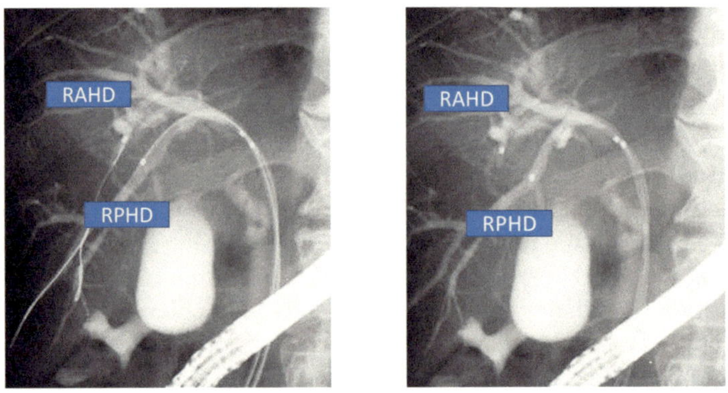

Figure 3.
Biliary imaging (ERCP) findings showed tumor invasion to the junction of the RAHD (right anterior hepatic duct) and RPHD right posterior hepatic duct (Bismuth-type IV). Insertion of ENBD tubes into anterior and posterior intrahepatic bile ducts.

type I and II HCCA, it is a popular opinion that endoscopic biliary drainage (EBD) is preferred over PTBD as it is rapid and moderately minimal invasive procedure [41].

Nevertheless, in patients with advanced and unopenable hilar malignancies including Bismuth types III and IV, it is indistinct if one method is superior to the other. Research have shown mixed results equating both these approaches [24, 31, 44–47]. In case of Bismuth type III and IV HCCA [48], numerous occasion of biliary decompression and drainage are needed. Even though several or bilateral ENBD is competent and carried out in certain determined conditions, three or more stenting only with regards to an endoscopic approach might be challenging to sustain adequate biliary drainage [39].

Cherqui et al. revealed the operative outcomes of 20 biliary cancer sufferers who gone through major hepatobiliary resection devoid of preoperative biliary drainage; the postoperative morbidity was substantially greater within the jaundiced patients, as the liver failure rate was 5% postoperatively, and fatality rate was recorded within the identical scenarios [49]. Besides PTBD, ERBD works extremely well as the preliminary treatment approach to strengthen obstructive jaundice in patients with unresectable HCCA if there's an extended time period of drainage patency following an effective drainage [44].

A latest multi intuitional retrospective analysis from Japan revealed that there are not considerable benefits of ENBD over EBS because the preliminary PBD for resectable hilar malignant biliary obstruction. On the other hand, the technical rate of success of preoperative ENBD was higher. Its re-intervention rate had not been diminutive and unexpected re-intervention was confederated with a poor prognosis in resected hilar biliary obstruction [50]. Authors quoted that [50]; ENBD for hilar biliary obstruction currently requires re-interventions, equally in the planned and unexpected way. It would need additional research in order to strengthen safety and efficiency of ENBD in those patients.

3. Portal vein embolization (PVE)

PVE and PBD are the two commonly used approaches to improve the FLR while preparing of major hepatectomy. According to our point of view ipsilateral portal vein occlusion along with the tumor with it could result in contralateral lobe hypertrophy. Preoperative PVE is actually performed to review the episode while planning for surgical procedure. In the event, FRL is not adequate for resection, PVE could be the conventional interposition to improve the volume of the FRL. Any local hemodynamic alterations could cause discharge of a varieties of growth factors and interleukins and that could possibly cause the hypertrophy of nonembolized hepatic lobe.

Within a CT volumetric review pre-operative PVE commonly offers somewhere around 10% of volume improvement in the FRL in contrast to 10% volume reduction in the embolized liver to get resected 2 weeks following PVE [51, 52]. Another study with PHC patients revealed that the FRL volume of less than 40% and liver function lesser than 2.7%/min/m^2 is the cutoff point for proceeding with PVE [38] . There is no need of biliary drainage within the embolized lobe without cholangitis, considering that there actually has a synergistic impact with unilateral cholestasis on the hypertrophy response on the non-embolized lobe. Over 3 weeks, following PVE, CT volumetric analysis and HBS should be replicated and reevaluated. Research showed that functional enhancement takes place more quickly than the volume level, implying that a reduced waiting time right up until resection can be done [53]. Within the series by Nagoya group from Japan revealed that PVE may enhance the operative outcomes of PHC [54]. PVE is recognized as a secure technique by having 2.2% of morbidity rate. Most commonly encountered complications are hemobilia, hematoma, septicemia, embolization material dislodgement and could consequently leads to thrombosis within the FRL [55].

Olthof et al. [56]; appraised the occurrence of postoperative liver failure in a collective succession of two European centers focused in PHC. They have recommended the risk score for PVE based upon FRL volume. It was coupled with jaundice at presentation, preoperative cholangitis and preoperative bilirubin level > 50 μmol/L [56]. PVE preceding to hepatectomy enables resection in the sufferer to advanced primary hepatobiliary tumors and insufficient FLR, with higher long-term survival [57]. Faster tumor development owing to PVE does not appear to impact the endurance to PHC patients [57, 58]. PVE, nonetheless, determine the resection of lobe and whenever newest findings that could need to have an alteration of approach, this can't be changed. During the waiting period if disease advancement occurs and inoperability ensues by the atrophy-hypertrophy reaction balances, extensive liver volume and its overall performance continued to be unaffected [38].

Having said that, the endurance with the atrophied, contaminated liver lobe might be associated with unwanted side-effects. For instance, liver abscess may further complicate the palliative management of the sufferer who commonly requires the repetitive procedures with stents [59]. Further embolization of (quadrate lobe) while preparing of extended right hemi hepatectomy is undoubtedly an alternative with regards to the targeted increment of FRL volume should be achieved. As a consequence, the left portal vein to quadrate lobes is occluded together with embolization of the right portal system. The strategy is complicated and needs a highly skilled interventional radiologist given that accessibility to left portal venous system can provide further injury risk. Backflow and dislodgement of embolization material in the left venous system may result in thrombosis in the portal veins offering the FRL. Additionally, to diminish these hazards, partially embolization of just segment 4a can be carried out [55, 60].

4. Surgical resection

Surgery provides the only opportunity of remedy in affected individuals with PHC. Surgical resection is depending upon the anatomical position and tumor and corresponding vessels and bile duct within the hepatic duct confluence. The operative consequences continue to be inadequate as a result of maximum recurrence [61]. The purposes of surgical procedures for PHC are to attain an R0 resection coupled with regional lymph nodes resection. Most often extrahepatic biliary duct resection with extended hepatectomy is mandatory based on the tumor location and its proximal extension on the segmental biliary ducts. In PHC, most often concomitant vascular resections and reconstruction are needed in order to achieve the negative margin. Our latest research implies that count of positive lymph nodes much better anticipates survival following surgical resection compared to lymph node resection in extrahepatic cholangiocarcinoma, given that lymph node assessment is enough [62]. Substantial number of lymph nodes, resection is justified for appropriate staging of nodal ailment. We firmly assume that comprehensive localized lymphadenectomy definitely seems to be required for effective resection of extrahepatic cholangiocarcinoma [62].

As the tumor ordinarily triggers biliary obstruction that is why hepatectomy in PHC is related to have high postoperative morbidity. PBD can be cast-off to generate a less hazardous setting in advance of surgical procedures, but biliary drainage might be detrimental when extreme drainage-related complications worsen the patients' condition or enhance the potential risk of postoperative morbidity [35].

Surgical resection is definitely the only possible curative remedy for HCCA; Bile duct resection in conjunction with significant hepatectomy could be the conventional treatment for HCCA. This treatment technique accomplishes an increased cure rate compared to that with bile duct resection alone [63]. While witnessing and assessing imaging reports, it is very imperative to comprehend three-dimensional fashion of the tumor locations and vascular and biliary involvement. The tumor expands across the left and right biliary ducts or in anterior and posterior course into the S4 or S1, correspondingly [38].

The Japanese institutes from the Nagoya were being the first one to demonstrate within the early 90s, that the intense strategy ended in much better long-term survival. The outcomes demonstrate that extreme surgical procedure of HCCA provides excellent consequences by having an adequate fatality rate [64]. Nevertheless, pursuing these guidelines, radical resection consists of hepatectomy or extended hemihepatectomy together with S4 and also the caudate lobe. Complete lymphadenectomy along with hepatoduodenal ligament and excision of the portal vein bifurcation should be done whenever required [65]. Approaches to optimize liver function as well as minimize removing functional liver parenchyma was connected with a reduction in fatality rate (7%) although an endeavor extended resection for HCCA by having an R0 resection rate of 92% [65].

Pathological study of the biliary ducts is carried out to substantiate radicality within the ductal level. The level of biliary resection could be expanded in the event of existence residual tumor in the resection margin. Survival was even worse within those patients as compared to the patient that had a preliminary free margin [66].

However, the segment one bile ducts typically drain within the left hepatic duct. Nevertheless, it could drain into any section of the hepatic duct confluence. These ducts are likely to be intricate by tumor concomitantly. Since 1998, authors routinely performing S1 resection en bloc coupled with extended hemihepatectomy and their results showed the substantial rates of R0 resections, and having an enhanced survival rate [67].

First of all, there is close proximity of the location of the biliary confluence and hepatoduodenal ligament in such circumstances the right sided liver resection enables additional comprehensive tumor margin. Quite often the right sided hepatic duct is normally shorter or lesser than 1 cm in length. In few instances it is missing in case existence of three confluences within the hepatic ducts. However, the left sided hepatic duct has a comparatively long and conventional course until attaining the left portal vein and splitting off into segments two and three hepatic ducts [68].

Consequently, malignancies that occupy the right intrahepatic ducts and perhaps the segment 4 in case of Bismuth-Corlette type IIIa-IV tumors. In such instances extended right hemihepatectomy should be considered. The potential drawback of such procedure is that segment two and three, are minor and quite smaller and therefore, in several patients right PVE is essential prior to extended right hemihepatectomy [38].

Tumors mainly relating to the left biliary duct, for instance, Bismuth-Corlette types IIIb-IV needs to have a left-sided approach. The main benefit of a left sided resection is usually that the remnant liver of the right liver normally has additional volume and resection could be expanded further to the right lobe of liver. Distinctly the volume of segments 6 plus 7 generally are higher than those of segments 2 and 3, which might lead the option of a right or left-sided technique [38]. An extended left hemihepatectomy adopting right hepatic vein with medial margin is technically challenging and dependent upon entanglement of the segment 8 biliary ducts.

5. Vascular resection and reconstruction

Portal vein resection and reconstruction (PVRR) prior to parenchymal transection are achievable in right-sided hepatectomies [69]. Neuhaus et al. described oncological advantages of hilar *en bloc* resection by means of 'no-touch' method for the handling of hilar cholangiocarcinoma [70]. In another study, the authors achieved PVRR through right-sided approach in case of decisive or extremely suspected invasion by the tumor to the portal vein [39]. Segmental resection along with end to end anastomosis is achievable in numerous instances. Segmental resection with autologous vein grafting is unusual in the right hepatectomy.

An autologous graft is required in the event of portal vein resection length is about 5–6 cm resection [39]. An external iliac vein is frequently used for an autologous graft for PVRR considering that the dimension of the harvested vein length is comparable to those of reconstruction. About 1/4th of the external iliac veins possess a valve, so normograde reconstruction of the portal vein is essential in order to avoid portal obstruction [39]. In portal vein reconstruction while utilizing an interposition graft, the proximal anastomosis is done prior to distal one. A distal anastomosis ought to be carried out following liberating the proximal clamp in order to inflate the anastomotic side. In left hepatectomies, PVRR ahead of liver resection take time and effort and apart from that exceptional, and segmental vein grafting is frequently necessary for reconstruction [39].

At our institute we use autologous vein grafting for PVRR (**Figure 4**). It depends upon the defect in the resected portal vein to get reconstructed, an immediate transverse suture can be used. Whenever we clamp the root of the left portal vein of umbilical part during right hepatectomy, we commonly evaluate the anticipated right-side hepatectomy to get achievable in terms of the PVRR. During an exceptional scenario where the bifurcation of the left lateral superior (P2) and umbilical portion of the left portal vein are intricate, and distal part of these portal branches are isolated, we commonly discretely fixed and obliquely resected from umbilical portion of the left portal vein to P2 during right hepatectomy. Most often an external iliac vein graft is essential for this type of portal vein resection as well as distinct performance is cast-off for the distal anastomosis to repair a big and oblique portal vein resection margin. The bilateral sides of the distal end of the graft are longitudinally incised to evolve the obliquely resected portal vein stump. In left-sided hepatectomies, the critical procedure necessitates the separation and fixing with the right posterior sectional or the right anterior portal vein. For the end to end anastomosis of the portal vein, a stay suture is positioned for both sides as well as an intraluminal method is ordinarily employed for the anastomosis of posterior wall. It is accompanied by anterior wall anastomosis with 6–0 prolene suture. Hepatobiliary surgeon should never be reluctant to carry out PVRR during hepatobiliary resection in case of an encouraging R0 resection in order to obtain a good outcome in locally advanced cholangiocarcinoma [39].

Right hemihepatectomy is superlative to achieve R0 resection in Bismuth type I or II with decisive or suspected involvement of right hepatic artery (RHA) [48, 71]. On the other hand, left hemihepatectomy with RHA resection and reconstruction is probably the alternate approaches for sufferers with deprived liver functional reserve [39]. An even additional intense strategy to patients with advanced predominant perihilar cholangiocarcinoma in the left side has now been utilized via trisegmentectomy by using RHA resection and reconstruction with or without simultaneous PVRR [72].

Whenever there is the need of concurrent vascular reconstruction, generally portal vein reconstruction must come before hepatic arterial reconstruction (**Figures 5** and **6**). Exactly where arterial reconstruction doesn't seem possible,

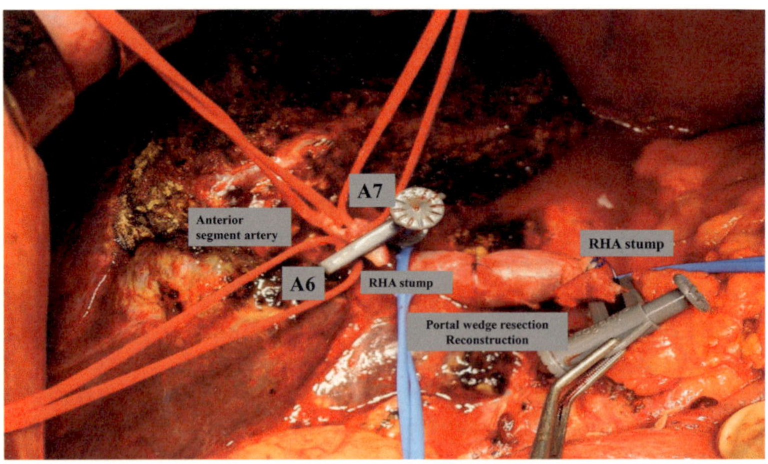

Figure 4.
Intra-operative illustrations of portal vein and right hepatic artery reconstruction.

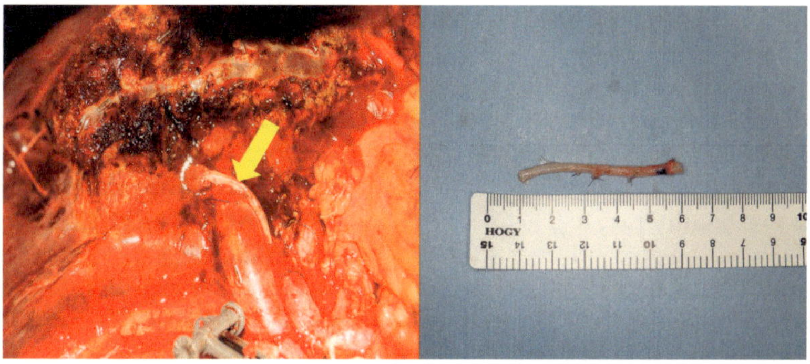

Figure 5.
Right hepatic artery reconstruction by using left radial artery (yellow arrow).

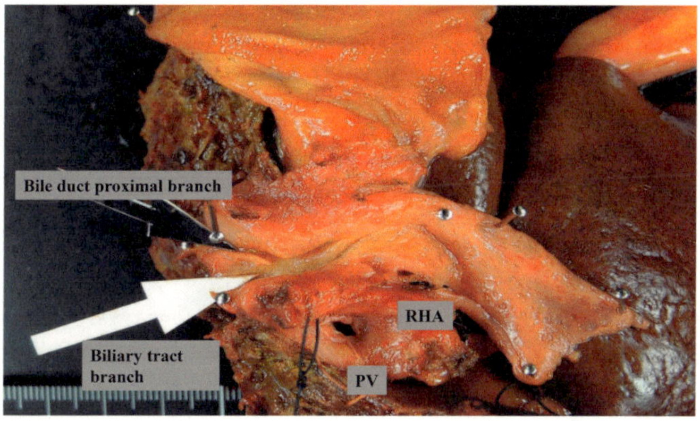

Figure 6.
Post-operative specimen illustrating the tumor invasion to the proximal branch and biliary tract including right hepatic artery and portal vein.

arterioportal shunting can be done by arterialization of the portal vein [73]. Side-to-oblique anastomosis is achieved between the common hepatic artery and the main portal vein, in order to avoid additional portal hypertension. Transcatheter arterial embolization of the common hepatic artery is conducted approximately 3 weeks right after surgical procedure. It could possibly evade liver infarction or abscess within the liver resulting in postoperative hepatic failure. Nevertheless, portal vein arterialization is phenomenal and also the ultimate disestablished alternative [39]. Adequate arterial perfusion is indispensable for the proper function of the remnant liver parenchyma. The left hepatic artery (LHA) cross transversely to the medial part of hepatoduodenal ligament and has significantly less risk for tumor engrossment.

The RHA having its right anterior and posterior branches is most often penetrated by tumor. Conducting a left or right arterial resection is frequently determined with the facet of the liver and the location where the branches of hepatic artery are free from the tumor. In PHC primarily relating to the left liver, extended or left hemihepatectomy with concomitant RHA resection is sometimes difficult in order to achieve tumor free margin. Intrahepatic distal stump for arterial reconstruction should be considered particularly when tumor mass is considerable. Micro surgical approaches are often employed to develop a risk-free anastomosis with the right posterior branch of the right hepatic artery in these instances (**Figure 5**). In Nagoya Japan, this complicated approach was associated with a fatality rate of 2% along with 30% of 5-year survival rate in advanced cholangiocarcinoma patients [72].

6. ALPPS for perihilar cholangiocarcinoma

Associating liver partition and portal vein ligation for staged hepatectomy (ALPPS) has become unveiled as a novel approach in liver surgery that causes speedy FLR hypertrophy assessed in liver volume and therefore, enables extensive resections. The initial report on the international ALPPS registry implemented and shown a deduction of fatality rate to 9% in 202 patients [74]. The foremost 25 patients series, explained the possibility of ALPPS to offer therapeutic resection primary or secondary advanced hepatic tumors, nevertheless, mortality rate was 12% [75].

Within one study, authors established that operative procedure of PHC employing ALPPS triggered a 48% mortality rate within 90 days. Coordinated sufferers that went through resection without having ALPPS had 28% mortality when compared with ALPPS (48%) patients, nevertheless, the main variance failed to achieve statistical importance [76].

Mortality resulting resection of PHC has been stated to vary from 5 to 18% in high volume centers [77–79]. PHC patient who was handled with ALPPS is highly recommended as very high risk patients and really should be in contrast to suitable risky controls. Having said that, along with the higher perils associated with ALPPS compared to the lower hazards of PVE, it could be much better to carry out a controlled PVE as the starting point rather than straight-up ALPPS. When it comes to inadequate hypertrophy, ALPPS could possibly be thought to be the last measure even though ALPPS-induced hypertrophy doesn't appear to be prone to prior PVE, most often designated as eventually salvage ALPPS [80]. Additionally, PHC sufferers have generally suffered with cholestasis, which hinders the restorative capability [81]. Consequently, the high re-forming response brought by ALPPS hypothetically may gain advantage to PHC patients. A disadvantage to PVE in the context of PHC is usually that long term embolization doesn't allow an intra-operative alteration of resection strategy, i.e. left to right or vice versa hepatectomy dependent upon intra-operative results [82].

ALPPS has got the advantages how the final choice to continue is usually obtained through the procedure. Nevertheless, the functional valuation on the speedy boost in liver volume noticed following phase one in ALPPS requires additional clinical evaluation [76]. According the latest study it has been recommended do not to consider ALPPS in PHC and one should relatively contemplate for PVE with selective embolization of the left portal vein to segment 4 for expansion of FRL volume in patients necessitating right trisegmentectomy [38]. When ALPPS is considered for PHC, the procedures needed to be carried out in specialized centers with substantial experience. On the other hand, depending on the existing details, PHC for ALPPS just isn't encouraged [76].

7. Summary

The management of PHC is complicated and needs close multidisciplinary team in order to gauze the preoperative planning for biliary drainage and determine the indications of operability. Imaging modalities such a MRCP could provide an additional assistance for tumor location. Patients with PHC usually presents with features of biliary issues, obstruction of biliary tract and jaundice. Biliary decompression is much-debated issue at present. We firmly believe that ENBD could a best modality for biliary decompression. Additional research is mandatory to validate this contentious issue. It is well known that obstructive jaundice hinders liver regeneration, biliary drainage remains recommended in the case of a small FLR and subsequently it could provide the likelihood of surgical resection. PVE is usually an extensively recognized interventional technique to enhance FRL volume and overall performance just before starting major liver resection. This approach of liver enlargement is particularly of great benefit in sufferers with PHC who are required extensive liver resection in pre-damaged livers.

The most significant prognostic factor for long-term survival of PHC is R0 in the hilar tumor with lymph node resection. In skilled and expertise hands, even Bismuth-Corlette type IV tumors could be resected with curative intent. R0 resection necessitates an aggressive operative technique encompassing hilar resection combined with extended liver resection, typically associated with vascular resection and reconstructions. The main advantages of en bloc, resection of the portal vein bifurcation is not yet determined. While it's remained associated with substantial morbidity and fatality rate, a hostile operative strategy adjacent to extended liver resection, regional lymphadenectomy and PVVR increase the only possibility of long-term survival.

Author details

Pankaj Prasoon, Kohei Miura, Kizuki Yuza, Yuki Hirose, Jun Sakata and Toshifumi Wakai*
Division of Digestive and General Surgery, Niigata University Graduate School of Medical and Dental Sciences, Niigata City, Japan

*Address all correspondence to: wakait@med.niigata-u.ac.jp

References

[1] Gatto M, Alvaro D. New insights on cholangiocarcinoma. World Journal of Gastrointestinal Oncology. 2010;**2**(3):136-145

[2] Bismuth H, Nakache R, Diamond T. Management strategies in resection for hilar cholangiocarcinoma. Annals of Surgery. 1992;**215**(1):31-38

[3] Khan SA, Thomas HC, Davidson BR, Taylor-Robinson SD. Cholangiocarcinoma. Lancet (London, England). 2005;**366**(9493):1303-1314

[4] Watanapa P, Watanapa WB. Liver fluke-associated cholangiocarcinoma. The British Journal of Surgery. 2002;**89**(8):962-970

[5] Shaib YH, El-Serag HB, Nooka AK, Thomas M, Brown TD, Patt YZ, et al. Risk factors for intrahepatic and extrahepatic cholangiocarcinoma: A hospital-based case-control study. The American Journal of Gastroenterology. 2007;**102**(5):1016-1021

[6] Walker NJ, Crockett PW, Nyska A, Brix AE, Jokinen MP, Sells DM, et al. Dose-additive carcinogenicity of a defined mixture of "dioxin-like compounds". Environmental Health Perspectives. 2005;**113**(1):43-48

[7] Shaib Y, El-Serag HB. The epidemiology of cholangiocarcinoma. Seminars in Liver Disease. 2004;**24**(2): 115-125

[8] Nimura Y, Hayakawa N, Kamiya J, Kondo S, Shionoya S. Hepatic segmentectomy with caudate lobe resection for bile duct carcinoma of the hepatic hilus. World Journal of Surgery. 1990;**14**(4):535-543; discussion 44

[9] Parodi A, Fisher D, Giovannini M, Baron T, Conio M. Endoscopic management of hilar cholangiocarcinoma. Nature Reviews Gastroenterology & Hepatology. 2012;**9**(2):105-112

[10] Wetter LA, Ring EJ, Pellegrini CA, Way LW. Differential diagnosis of sclerosing cholangiocarcinomas of the common hepatic duct (Klatskin tumors). American Journal of Surgery. 1991;**161**(1):57-62; discussion-3

[11] Shigeta H, Nagino M, Kamiya J, Uesaka K, Sano T, Yamamoto H, et al. Bacteremia after hepatectomy: An analysis of a single-center, 10-year experience with 407 patients. Langenbeck's Archives of Surgery. 2002;**387**(3-4):117-124

[12] Dixon JM, Armstrong CP, Duffy SW, Davies GC. Factors affecting morbidity and mortality after surgery for obstructive jaundice: A review of 373 patients. Gut. 1983;**24**(9):845-852

[13] Blamey SL, Fearon KC, Gilmour WH, Osborne DH, Carter DC. Prediction of risk in biliary surgery. The British Journal of Surgery. 1983;**70**(9):535-538

[14] Nimura Y. Preoperative biliary drainage before resection for cholangiocarcinoma (pro). HPB: The Official Journal of the International Hepato Pancreato Biliary Association. 2008;**10**(2):130-133

[15] Kawasaki S, Imamura H, Kobayashi A, Noike T, Miwa S, Miyagawa S. Results of surgical resection for patients with hilar bile duct cancer: Application of extended hepatectomy after biliary drainage and hemihepatic portal vein embolization. Annals of Surgery. 2003;**238**(1):84-92

[16] Maguchi H, Takahashi K, Katanuma A, Osanai M, Nakahara K, Matuzaki S, et al. Preoperative biliary drainage for hilar cholangiocarcinoma. Journal

of Hepato-Biliary-Pancreatic Surgery. 2007;**14**(5):441-446

[17] Paik WH, Loganathan N, Hwang JH. Preoperative biliary drainage in hilar cholangiocarcinoma: When and how? World Journal of Gastrointestinal Endoscopy. 2014;**6**(3):68-73

[18] Pitt HA, Gomes AS, Lois JF, Mann LL, Deutsch LS, Longmire WP Jr. Does preoperative percutaneous biliary drainage reduce operative risk or increase hospital cost? Annals of Surgery. 1985;**201**(5):545-553

[19] Lau SH, Lau WY. Current therapy of hilar cholangiocarcinoma. Hepatobiliary & Pancreatic Diseases International: HBPD INT. 2012;**11**(1):12-17

[20] Belghiti J, Hiramatsu K, Benoist S, Massault P, Sauvanet A, Farges O. Seven hundred forty-seven hepatectomies in the 1990s: An update to evaluate the actual risk of liver resection. Journal of the American College of Surgeons. 2000;**191**(1):38-46

[21] Gundry SR, Strodel WE, Knol JA, Eckhauser FE, Thompson NW. Efficacy of preoperative biliary tract decompression in patients with obstructive jaundice. Archives of Surgery (Chicago, Ill: 1960). 1984;**119**(6):703-708

[22] Kim KM, Park JW, Lee JK, Lee KH, Lee KT, Shim SG. A comparison of preoperative biliary drainage methods for perihilar cholangiocarcinoma: Endoscopic versus percutaneous transhepatic biliary drainage. Gut and Liver. 2015;**9**(6):791-799

[23] van der Gaag NA, Kloek JJ, de Castro SM, Busch OR, van Gulik TM, Gouma DJ. Preoperative biliary drainage in patients with obstructive jaundice: History and current status. Journal of Gastrointestinal Surgery: Official Journal of the Society for Surgery of the Alimentary Tract. 2009;**13**(4):814-820

[24] Kloek JJ, van der Gaag NA, Aziz Y, Rauws EA, van Delden OM, Lameris JS, et al. Endoscopic and percutaneous preoperative biliary drainage in patients with suspected hilar cholangiocarcinoma. Journal of Gastrointestinal Surgery: Official Journal of the Society for Surgery of the Alimentary Tract. 2010;**14**(1):119-125

[25] Kawakami H, Kuwatani M, Onodera M, Haba S, Eto K, Ehira N, et al. Endoscopic nasobiliary drainage is the most suitable preoperative biliary drainage method in the management of patients with hilar cholangiocarcinoma. Journal of Gastroenterology. 2011;**46**(2):242-248

[26] Hwang S, Song GW, Ha TY, Lee YJ, Kim KH, Ahn CS, et al. Reappraisal of percutaneous transhepatic biliary drainage tract recurrence after resection of perihilar bile duct cancer. World Journal of Surgery. 2012;**36**(2):379-385

[27] Takahashi Y, Nagino M, Nishio H, Ebata T, Igami T, Nimura Y. Percutaneous transhepatic biliary drainage catheter tract recurrence in cholangiocarcinoma. The British Journal of Surgery. 2010;**97**(12):1860-1866

[28] Mansfield SD, Barakat O, Charnley RM, Jaques BC, O'Suilleabhain CB, Atherton PJ, et al. Management of hilar cholangiocarcinoma in the North of England: Pathology, treatment, and outcome. World Journal of Gastroenterology. 2005;**11**(48):7625-7630

[29] Goenka MK, Goenka U. Palliation: Hilar cholangiocarcinoma. World Journal of Hepatology. 2014;**6**(8):559-569

[30] Rerknimitr R, Angsuwatcharakon P, Ratanachu-ek T, Khor CJ, Ponnudurai R, Moon JH, et al. Asia-Pacific consensus recommendations for endoscopic and interventional management of hilar cholangiocarcinoma. Journal of

Gastroenterology and Hepatology. 2013;**28**(4):593-607

[31] Paik WH, Park YS, Hwang JH, Lee SH, Yoon CJ, Kang SG, et al. Palliative treatment with self-expandable metallic stents in patients with advanced type III or IV hilar cholangiocarcinoma: A percutaneous versus endoscopic approach. Gastrointestinal Endoscopy. 2009;**69**(1):55-62

[32] Rerknimitr R, Kladcharoen N, Mahachai V, Kullavanijaya P. Result of endoscopic biliary drainage in hilar cholangiocarcinoma. Journal of Clinical Gastroenterology. 2004;**38**(6):518-523

[33] Moole H, Dharmapuri S, Duvvuri A, Dharmapuri S, Boddireddy R, Moole V, et al. Endoscopic versus percutaneous biliary drainage in palliation of advanced malignant hilar obstruction: A meta-analysis and systematic review. 2016;**2016**:4726078

[34] Celotti A, Solaini L, Montori G, Coccolini F, Tognali D, Baiocchi G. Preoperative biliary drainage in hilar cholangiocarcinoma: Systematic review and meta-analysis. European Journal of Surgical Oncology: The Journal of the European Society of Surgical Oncology and the British Association of Surgical Oncology. 2017;**43**(9):1628-1635

[35] Wiggers JK, Coelen RJ, Rauws EA, van Delden OM, van Eijck CH, de Jonge J, et al. Preoperative endoscopic versus percutaneous transhepatic biliary drainage in potentially resectable perihilar cholangiocarcinoma (DRAINAGE trial): Design and rationale of a randomized controlled trial. BMC Gastroenterology. 2015;**15**:20

[36] Jo JH, Chung MJ, Han DH, Park JY, Bang S, Park SW, et al. Best options for preoperative biliary drainage in patients with Klatskin tumors. Surgical Endoscopy. 2017;**31**(1):422-429

[37] Komaya K, Ebata T, Yokoyama Y, Igami T, Sugawara G, Mizuno T, et al. Verification of the oncologic inferiority of percutaneous biliary drainage to endoscopic drainage: A propensity score matching analysis of resectable perihilar cholangiocarcinoma. Surgery. 2017;**161**(2):394-404

[38] Rassam F, Roos E, van Lienden KP, van Hooft JE, Klumpen HJ, van Tienhoven G, et al. Modern work-up and extended resection in perihilar cholangiocarcinoma: The AMC experience. Langenbeck's Archives of Surgery. 2018;**403**(3):289-307

[39] Sano T, Shimizu Y, Senda Y, Kinoshita T, Nimura Y. Assessing resectability in cholangiocarcinoma. Hepatic Oncology. 2014;**1**(1):39-51

[40] Sewnath ME, Karsten TM, Prins MH, Rauws EJ, Obertop H, Gouma DJ. A meta-analysis on the efficacy of preoperative biliary drainage for tumors causing obstructive jaundice. Annals of Surgery. 2002;**236**(1):17-27

[41] Kawashima H, Itoh A, Ohno E, Itoh Y, Ebata T, Nagino M, et al. Preoperative endoscopic nasobiliary drainage in 164 consecutive patients with suspected perihilar cholangiocarcinoma: A retrospective study of efficacy and risk factors related to complications. Annals of Surgery. 2013;**257**(1):121-127

[42] Ratti F, Cipriani F, Ferla F, Catena M, Paganelli M, Aldrighetti LA. Hilar cholangiocarcinoma: Preoperative liver optimization with multidisciplinary approach. Toward a better outcome. World Journal of Surgery. 2013;**37**(6):1388-1396

[43] Kanai M, Nimura Y, Kamiya J, Kondo S, Nagino M, Miyachi M, et al. Preoperative intrahepatic segmental cholangitis in patients with advanced carcinoma involving the hepatic hilus. Surgery. 1996;**119**(5):498-504

[44] Choi J, Ryu JK, Lee SH, Ahn DW, Hwang JH, Kim YT, et al. Biliary drainage for obstructive jaundice caused by unresectable hepatocellular carcinoma: The endoscopic versus percutaneous approach. Hepatobiliary & Pancreatic Diseases International: HBPD INT. 2012;**11**(6):636-642

[45] Saluja SS, Gulati M, Garg PK, Pal H, Pal S, Sahni P, et al. Endoscopic or percutaneous biliary drainage for gallbladder cancer: A randomized trial and quality of life assessment. Clinical Gastroenterology and Hepatology: The Official Clinical Practice Journal of the American Gastroenterological Association. 2008;**6**(8):944-50.e3

[46] Pinol V, Castells A, Bordas JM, Real MI, Llach J, Montana X, et al. Percutaneous self-expanding metal stents versus endoscopic polyethylene endoprostheses for treating malignant biliary obstruction: Randomized clinical trial. Radiology. 2002;**225**(1):27-34

[47] Born P, Rosch T, Bruhl K, Sandschin W, Weigert N, Ott R, et al. Long-term outcome in patients with advanced hilar bile duct tumors undergoing palliative endoscopic or percutaneous drainage. Zeitschrift fur Gastroenterologie. 2000;**38**(6):483-489

[48] Bismuth H, Corlette MB. Intrahepatic cholangioenteric anastomosis in carcinoma of the hilus of the liver. Surgery, Gynecology & Obstetrics. 1975;**140**(2):170-178

[49] Cherqui D, Benoist S, Malassagne B, Humeres R, Rodriguez V, Fagniez PL. Major liver resection for carcinoma in jaundiced patients without preoperative biliary drainage. Archives of Surgery (Chicago, Ill: 1960). 2000;**135**(3):302-308

[50] Nakai Y, Yamamoto R, Matsuyama M, Sakai Y, Takayama Y, Ushio J, et al. Multicenter study of endoscopic preoperative biliary drainage for malignant hilar biliary obstruction: E-POD hilar study. Journal of Gastroenterology and Hepatology. 2018;**33**(5):1146-1153

[51] Makuuchi M, Thai BL, Takayasu K, Takayama T, Kosuge T, Gunven P, et al. Preoperative portal embolization to increase safety of major hepatectomy for hilar bile duct carcinoma: A preliminary report. Surgery. 1990;**107**(5):521-527

[52] Nagino M, Nimura Y, Kamiya J, Kondo S, Uesaka K, Kin Y, et al. Changes in hepatic lobe volume in biliary tract cancer patients after right portal vein embolization. Hepatology (Baltimore, Md). 1995;**21**(2):434-439

[53] de Graaf W, van Lienden KP, van den Esschert JW, Bennink RJ, van Gulik TM. Increase in future remnant liver function after preoperative portal vein embolization. The British Journal of Surgery. 2011;**98**(6):825-834

[54] Nagino M, Ebata T, Yokoyama Y, Igami T, Sugawara G, Takahashi Y, et al. Evolution of surgical treatment for perihilar cholangiocarcinoma: A single-center 34-year review of 574 consecutive resections. Annals of Surgery. 2013;**258**(1):129-140

[55] van Gulik TM, van den Esschert JW, de Graaf W, van Lienden KP, Busch OR, Heger M, et al. Controversies in the use of portal vein embolization. Digestive Surgery. 2008;**25**(6):436-444

[56] Olthof PB, Wiggers JK, Groot Koerkamp B, Coelen RJ, Allen PJ, Besselink MG, et al. Postoperative liver failure risk score: Identifying patients with resectable perihilar cholangiocarcinoma who can benefit from portal vein embolization. Journal of the American College of Surgeons. 2017;**225**(3):387-394

[57] Glantzounis GK, Tokidis E, Basourakos SP, Ntzani EE, Lianos GD, Pentheroudakis G. The role of portal

vein embolization in the surgical management of primary hepatobiliary cancers. A systematic review. European Journal of Surgical Oncology: The Journal of the European Society of Surgical Oncology and the British Association of Surgical Oncology. 2017;**43**(1):32-41

[58] Hayashi S, Baba Y, Ueno K, Nakajo M, Kubo F, Ueno S, et al. Acceleration of primary liver tumor growth rate in embolized hepatic lobe after portal vein embolization. Acta Radiologica (Stockholm, Sweden: 1987). 2007;**48**(7):721-727

[59] Huisman F, Cieslak KP, van Lienden KP, Bennink RJ, van Gulik TM. Liver related complications in unresectable disease after portal vein embolization. Hepatobiliary Surgery and Nutrition. 2017;**6**(6):379-386

[60] van Lienden KP, van den Esschert JW, de Graaf W, Bipat S, Lameris JS, van Gulik TM, et al. Portal vein embolization before liver resection: A systematic review. Cardiovascular and Interventional Radiology. 2013;**36**(1):25-34

[61] Wakai T, Sakata J. Surgical management of carcinoma in situ at ductal resection margins in patients with extrahepatic cholangiocarcinoma. 2018;**2**(5):359-366

[62] Sakata J, Wakai T, Matsuda Y, Ohashi T, Hirose Y, Ichikawa H, et al. Comparison of number versus ratio of positive lymph nodes in the assessment of lymph node status in extrahepatic cholangiocarcinoma. Annals of Surgical Oncology. 2016;**23**(1):225-234

[63] Ito F, Agni R, Rettammel RJ, Been MJ, Cho CS, Mahvi DM, et al. Resection of hilar cholangiocarcinoma: Concomitant liver resection decreases hepatic recurrence. Annals of Surgery. 2008;**248**(2):273-279

[64] Nishio H, Nagino M, Nimura Y. Surgical management of hilar cholangiocarcinoma: The Nagoya experience. HPB: The Official Journal of the International Hepato Pancreato Biliary Association. 2005;**7**(4):259-262

[65] van Gulik TM, Ruys AT, Busch OR, Rauws EA, Gouma DJ. Extent of liver resection for hilar cholangiocarcinoma (Klatskin tumor): How much is enough? Digestive Surgery. 2011;**28**(2):141-147

[66] Wiggers JK, Groot Koerkamp B, Coelen RJ, Rauws EA, Schattner MA, Nio CY, et al. Preoperative biliary drainage in perihilar cholangiocarcinoma: Identifying patients who require percutaneous drainage after failed endoscopic drainage. Endoscopy. 2015;**47**(12):1124-1131

[67] Dinant S, Gerhards MF, Busch ORC, Obertop H, Gouma DJ, Van Gulik TM. The importance of complete excision of the caudate lobe in resection of hilar cholangiocarcinoma. HPB: The Official Journal of the International Hepato Pancreato Biliary Association. 2005;**7**(4):263-267

[68] Bismuth H. Surgical anatomy and anatomical surgery of the liver. World Journal of Surgery. 1982;**6**(1):3-9

[69] Kondo S, Katoh H, Hirano S, Ambo Y, Tanaka E, Okushiba S. Portal vein resection and reconstruction prior to hepatic dissection during right hepatectomy and caudate lobectomy for hepatobiliary cancer. The British Journal of Surgery. 2003;**90**(6):694-697

[70] Neuhaus P, Thelen A, Jonas S, Puhl G, Denecke T, Veltzke-Schlieker W, et al. Oncological superiority of hilar en bloc resection for the treatment of hilar cholangiocarcinoma. Annals of Surgical Oncology. 2012;**19**(5):1602-1608

[71] Ikeyama T, Nagino M, Oda K, Ebata T, Nishio H, Nimura Y. Surgical approach to Bismuth type I and II hilar

cholangiocarcinomas: Audit of 54 consecutive cases. Annals of Surgery. 2007;**246**(6):1052-1057

[72] Nagino M, Nimura Y, Nishio H, Ebata T, Igami T, Matsushita M, et al. Hepatectomy with simultaneous resection of the portal vein and hepatic artery for advanced perihilar cholangiocarcinoma: An audit of 50 consecutive cases. Annals of Surgery. 2010;**252**(1):115-123

[73] Kondo S, Hirano S, Ambo Y, Tanaka E, Kubota T, Katoh H. Arterioportal shunting as an alternative to microvascular reconstruction after hepatic artery resection. The British Journal of Surgery. 2004;**91**(2):248-251

[74] Schadde E, Ardiles V, Robles-Campos R, Malago M, Machado M, Hernandez-Alejandro R, et al. Early survival and safety of ALPPS: First report of the International ALPPS Registry. Annals of Surgery. 2014;**260**(5):829-836; discussion 36-8

[75] Schnitzbauer AA, Lang SA, Goessmann H, Nadalin S, Baumgart J, Farkas SA, et al. Right portal vein ligation combined with in situ splitting induces rapid left lateral liver lobe hypertrophy enabling 2-staged extended right hepatic resection in small-for-size settings. Annals of Surgery. 2012;**255**(3):405-414

[76] Olthof PB, Coelen RJS, Wiggers JK, Groot Koerkamp B, Malago M, Hernandez-Alejandro R, et al. High mortality after ALPPS for perihilar cholangiocarcinoma: Case-control analysis including the first series from the International ALPPS registry. HPB: The Official Journal of the International Hepato Pancreato Biliary Association. 2017;**19**(5):381-387

[77] Olthof PB, Coelen RJ, Wiggers JK, Besselink MG, Busch OR, van Gulik TM. External biliary drainage following major liver resection for perihilar cholangiocarcinoma: Impact on development of liver failure and biliary leakage. HPB: The Official Journal of the International Hepato Pancreato Biliary Association. 2016;**18**(4):348-353

[78] Kaiser GM, Paul A, Sgourakis G, Molmenti EP, Dechene A, Trarbach T, et al. Novel prognostic scoring system after surgery for Klatskin tumor. The American Surgeon. 2013;**79**(1):90-95

[79] DeOliveira ML, Cunningham SC, Cameron JL, Kamangar F, Winter JM, Lillemoe KD, et al. Cholangiocarcinoma: Thirty-one-year experience with 564 patients at a single institution. Annals of Surgery. 2007;**245**(5):755-762

[80] Bjornsson B, Gasslander T, Sandstrom P. In situ split of the liver when portal venous embolization fails to induce hypertrophy: A report of two cases. Case Reports in Surgery. 2013;**2013**:238675

[81] Yokoyama Y, Nagino M, Nimura Y. Mechanism of impaired hepatic regeneration in cholestatic liver. Journal of Hepato-Biliary-Pancreatic Surgery. 2007;**14**(2):159-166

[82] Donati M, Stavrou GA, van Gulik TM, Oldhafer KJ. Associating liver partition and portal vein ligation for staged hepatectomy for Klatskin tumours: Hinc sunt Leones! ANZ Journal of Surgery. 2015;**85**(1-2):3-4

Section 5

Distal Bile Duct Cancer

Chapter 6

Distal Cholangiocarcinoma

Ahmad Abdullah Madkhali and Faisal Al-alem

Abstract

Cholangiocarcinoma arises from the epithelial lining of the biliary tree. It accounts for approximately 3% of all gastrointestinal malignancies. This chapter looks at the new advances that have been made in the management of distal cholangiocarcinoma, based on a literature review. Diagnosis of the disease resides mainly in clinical presentation and radiological diagnosis and biopsy indicated in selected cases. Surgical resection is the main curative treatment for distal cholangiocarcinoma, and resectability of the tumor can now be assessed using multiple radiological imaging studies. Resection margins and lymph node invasion status are the two important prognostic factors after surgery. Pancreaticoduodenectomy is the standard surgical treatment of choice in distal cholangiocarcinoma; however, combined major vascular and hepatopancreaticoduodenectomy can be indicated in selected cases. Adjuvant therapy is clearly indicated after surgical resection with survival improvement, but optimal adjuvant treatment strategy has not yet been established.

Keywords: cholangiocarcinoma, bile duct cancer, pancreaticoduodenectomy

1. Introduction

Cholangiocarcinoma arises from the epithelial lining of the biliary tree. Given the biliary tree anatomical differences and diversity, biliary tree cancers are most commonly classified according to their location into intrahepatic and extrahepatic cholangiocarcinomas, which are further classified into perihilar and distal type. Over all, these malignancies account for approximately 3% of all gastrointestinal malignancies [1]. Perihilar cholangiocarcinoma accounts for 50% of them, followed by distal cholangiocarcinoma (40%), and the remainder is intrahepatic disease [2].

Cholangiocarcinoma can also be classified based on its macroscopic growth pattern into three types: mass-forming exophytic type, periductal infiltrative type, or intraductal polypoid type. For distal cholangiocarcinoma, the periductal infiltrative type is the most common macroscopic growth pattern identified [3].

2. Staging and survival

Over all, biliary malignancies have poor prognosis. Surgical resection is the mainstay of treatment and it is possible only for localized disease without distant spread. The resection rate of bile duct cancer is different based on its location, and distal bile duct cancer has the highest respectability rate among other types [4]. In distal bile duct cancer, patients usually manifest jaundice early in the disease course and likely seek medical care prior to metastasis development. Lymph node involvement, perineural invasion, lymphatic invasion, vascular invasion, and pancreatic invasion in addition to tumor depth of invasion are important prognostic factors and correlated with survival [5–8]. However, achieving negative resection margins is proposed to be the single most important predictor of survival [8]. The 8th AJCC UICC 2017 categorized cholangiocarcinoma based on its location in intrahepatic,

Primary tumor (T)			
T category	**T criteria**		
TX	Primary tumor cannot be assessed		
Tis	Carcinoma in situ/high-grade dysplasia		
T1	Tumor invades the bile duct wall with a depth less than 5 mm		
T2	Tumor invades the bile duct wall with a depth of 5–12 mm		
T3	Tumor invades the bile duct wall with a depth greater than 12 mm		
T4	Tumor involves the celiac axis, superior mesenteric artery, and/or common hepatic artery		
Regional lymph nodes (N)			
N category	**N criteria**		
NX	Regional lymph nodes cannot be assessed		
N0	No regional lymph node metastasis		
N1	Metastasis in one to three regional lymph nodes		
N2	Metastasis in four or more regional lymph nodes		
Distant metastasis (M)			
M category	**M criteria**		
M0	No distant metastasis		
M1	Distant metastasis		
Prognostic stage groups			
When T is...	**And N is...**	**And M is...**	**Then the stage group is...**
Tis	N0	M0	0
T1	N0	M0	I
T1	N1	M0	IIA
T1	N2	M0	IIIA
T2	N0	M0	IIA
T2	N1	M0	IIB
T2	N2	M0	IIIA
T3	N0	M0	IIB
T3	N1	M0	IIB
T3	N2	M0	IIIA
T4	N0	M0	IIIB
T4	N1	M0	IIIB
T4	N2	M0	IIIB
Any T	Any N	M1	IV

Table 1.
Distal bile duct cancer TNM staging AJCC UICC 2017 [12].

hilar, and distal type and provided separate staging system for each one. The recent changes in distal CBD cancer designated the T level according to the depth of invasion rather than invaded structures, and N stage would include the number of involved lymph nodes rather than being involved or not. N1 will be given for involvement of 1–3 lymph nodes and N2 for the involvement of 4 and more lymph nodes **Table 1**. These changes improved the survival stratification between the stages based on the TNM stage [9, 10]. The overall 5-year survival of stages I, II, and III was 59.0, 35.4, and 14.7%, respectively [10].

3. Clinical presentation and diagnosis

The typical presentation of distal cholangiocarcinoma is painless jaundice in patients in the 5th–7th decade of life, while 10% of patients will have cholangitis as their initial presentation. A total of 56% of patients will present with constitutional symptom of malignancy like anorexia, fatigue, and weight loss [11]. Serum biochemical testing will show cholestatic jaundice pattern with elevated alkaline phosphatase, gamma-glutamyl transpeptidase and bilirubin levels. CA 19-9 is a tumor marker used in the workup of bile duct cancer. It has low sensitivity and specificity for cholangiocarcinoma, and it can also be elevated in biliary obstruction of benign disease. CA 19-9 seems to be correlated with prognosis and stage of the disease [12, 13], but its role as a diagnostic test is limited.

Cross sectional, enhanced contrast imaging is essential diagnostic modality in patients with distal cholangiocarcinoma, and it should be obtained before biliary intervention since its accuracy will be diminished after stent as a result of decompression, image artifact, or as consequence of local complication to the biliary intervention [14, 15]. Cholangiocarcinoma may be seen as stricture (**Figure 1**) in periductal infiltrative type or mass forming lesion in intraductal polypoid type or exophytic type. High resolution CT can identify biliary dilatation, tumor extent, and its relationship with the vascular system and adjacent organ, anatomical variation, lymphadenopathy, and distant metastasis. Periductal infiltrative type may manifest as thickened bile duct wall, which is often seen on CT as hypoattenuated on portovenous and hyperattenuated on delayed phase [16, 17]. Magnetic resonance imaging (MRI) with magnetic resonance cholangiopancreatography (MRCP) is a noninvasive modality that is competent to provide cholangiography for assessing the extent of bile duct extension and considered the preferred imaging for the diagnosis of suspected cholangiocarcinoma. Utilizing the high soft tissue contrasts and multiplanar capability, it is better at detecting infiltrative ductal tumor and its

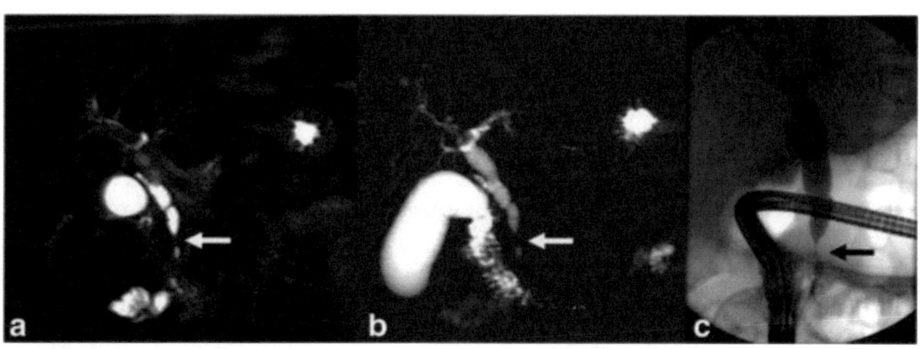

Figure 1.
Distal cholangiocarcinoma. Images showing narrowing segment in distal common bile duct (stricture) (arrow) with proximal biliary dilatation in coronal T2-weighted image (a), MRCP (b), and ERCP (c) [20].

local extent of tumor, biliary anatomy, invasion to surrounding structure, and liver metastasis. However, it is inferior to high resolution CT for vascular involvement and distant metastasis [18–21].Infiltrating periductal cholangiocarcinoma can be identified on MRI as irregular wall thickening of bile duct, with proximal biliary dilatation, which enhances gradually to peak on delayed image, while intraductal polypoid type is typically identified as enhancing intraductal mass with proximal biliary dilation [22, 23]. MRCP is an essential noninvasive cholangiography to evaluate the longitudinal tumor extension in the bile duct proximal and distal to the obstruction and provides valuable preoperative biliary mapping [24]. It has higher sensitivity, specificity, and accuracy in differentiating benign from malignant biliary obstruction compared to ERCP [24].

Cholangiocarcinoma can be evaluated also by direct cholangiography with endoscopic retrograde cholangiopancreatography (ERCP) (**Figure 1**) or percutaneous transhepatic cholangiography (PTC), which typically present as dominant stricture or filling defect. They can delineate biliary anatomy and determine the level of bile duct involvement, which will help to identify resectability and surgical planning. It also allows for bile sampling for brush cytology and relives the biliary obstruction. The diagnostic yield of cytology has a low sensitivity of 42% but a high specificity of 98% and a positive predictive value of 98% of patients who had cancers [25]. The sensitivity of brush cytology can be improved further more to 46–68% by using fluorescence in situ hybridization (FISH) to detect cancerous epithelial cells [26, 27]. EUS is an important diagnostic tool in the evaluation of distal biliary obstruction because it is very specific in predicting unresectability [28], and it is challenging some time to differentiate distal cholangiocarcinoma from other periampullary tumors based on other diagnostic modality. It helps to assess the extrahepatic biliary system, regional lymph node, and local extension to adjacent structure [24, 29]. It can also detect small lesions that were missed by another modality [28]. The sensitivity and specificity of EUS in detecting malignant biliary stricture are reported to be, in meta-analysis, 78 and 84%, respectively [30]. EUS also facilitates FNA cytology assessment which will increase the diagnostic yield of EUS. Recent meta-analysis found that EUS-FNA has a sensitivity of 80% and a specificity of 97% for diagnosing malignant biliary stricture [31].

The diagnostic algorithm is controversial in the literature, and it depends on institutional availability and experience of different diagnostic modalities. However, a general concept in evaluating distal cholangiocarcinoma is to determine tumor resectability, by assessing local extension of the tumor and its relationship with adjacent organs including vascular structure and presence of distant metastasis, and biliary tree mapping to assess longitudinal tumor extension. Cross-sectional, enhanced contrast imaging with MRI and/or CT with MRCP is the preferred diagnostic modality [32, 33] for assessing bile duct cancer. Direct cholangiography with ERCP/PTC is necessary in unresectable patients or in patients who need therapeutic intervention [33]. For patients with resectable disease, preoperative pathological diagnosis in not necessary [32, 33], especially in highly suspicious cases of malignant biliary obstruction, since diagnostic yield of preoperative tissue biopsy is low and cannot rule out malignancy. In patients with unresectable disease or when the diagnosis is not clear, then, biopsy is indicated. Serum IgG4 should also be considered if diagnosis is not clear because IgG4-associated cholangitis may present with jaundice and stricture, mimicking cholangiocarcinoma [33]. Preoperative biliary drainage is definitely indicated in patients with acute cholangitis or if patients will have delayed surgery for preoperative optimization [15, 24]. Preoperative routine drainage is not preferred owing to increased postoperative complication with no added benefit compared to no drainage [34, 35].

4. Surgical treatment

Surgical resection with curative intent is the only cure for distal cholangiocarcinoma. In most cases, pancreaticoduodenectomy is the surgical procedure for periampullary tumors, including distal cholangiocarcinoma. The goal of curative resection is to resect the tumor and regional lymph node with negative resection margin [36, 37]. Achieving a precise review of imaging to assess local extension of the tumor, lymph node, proximal ductal involvement, and presence of distant metastasis is an essential step in surgical planning to reach to the best outcome. The presence of peritoneal or distant metastasis (lung, liver, bone, or paraaortic lymph node) considered a contraindication for surgery [38, 39]. En-bloc major vascular resection may be necessary to achieve complete oncologic resection and does not preclude curative resection. Portal vein and/or hepatic artery resection and reconstruction are indicated if the tumor is locally advanced and invading them. Pancreaticoduodenectomy combined with vascular resection is reported to be a feasible technique with acceptable mortality, morbidity, and survival benefit [40].

Lymph node metastasis is an independent predictor for poor survival in distal cholangiocarcinoma [41]. Adequate lymphadenectomy for regional lymph node is important for complete oncologic resection, staging purpose, and planning of postoperative adjuvant therapy. Regional lymph node of distal bile duct is defined to be the lymph node along the porta hepatis, hepatic artery, anterior and posterior to the head of pancreas, and the lymph node along superior mesenteric artery [42].

Resection margin status of bile duct is highly correlated with survival in cholangiocarcinoma. Adequate assessment of the biliary system before any surgical planning is a critical step to achieve negative resection margin. Identification of the proximal extent of the disease helps to define the level of proximal resection and identify the patients who need a more extensive procedure to undergo preoperative optimization. Patients who have extensive periductal infiltration into the intrahepatic biliary duct may benefit from hepatopancreaticoduodenectomy (HPD) and should not be precluded from curative resection [33]. It is considered aggressive surgical resection for extrahepatic cholangiocarcinoma; however, with the improvement in surgical techniques and perioperative care, the postoperative mortality improved, compared to early experience, and it demonstrated favorable survival once the negative resection margin was achieved [43]. This procedure may be justified in well-selected and prepared patients, which may include perioperative biliary drainage and portal vein embolization to augment future liver remnant hypertrophy, with advanced cholangiocarcinoma [44]. Intraoperative frozen section of the proximal duct margin is required to assess margin status, and further re-resection is indicated when it is feasible to achieve negative resection margin. However, sometimes, the frozen section is repeatedly positive and no more extrahepatic bile duct to be excised, which conveys a challenging situation. If the frozen section report is carcinoma in situ, then no resection is required because it has comparable oncologic outcome with negative resection margin [45, 46], but if the frozen section is positive for invasive cancer, then unplanned hepatopancreaticoduodenectomy (HPD) may be indicated in selected cases. Minor or major central liver resection in this situation can help to achieve negative resection margin and preserve functional liver parenchyma, especially in those patients who are not well prepared for major hepatectomy, with no decreased long-term survival been reported in hilar cholangiocarcinoma literature. Left hepatectomy can also be an option in cases with left hepatic duct only involvement, because it reserves more future liver remnant in comparison to right hepatectomy or trisegmentectomy [47, 48]. However, it is a comorbid procedure, and risks and benefits should critically be evaluated and balanced before attempting liver resection in this situation.

After curative resection, the risk of recurrence dictates the need for additional treatment modality to improve disease-free and overall survival. The role of adjuvant therapy in cholangiocarcinoma is not yet agreed on because most of these studies combine different types of hepatobiliary cancers and nonrandomized studies. However, the available data, including randomized trial, showed survival benefit and suggested that chemotherapy can decrease the risk of distant recurrences while radiotherapy or chemoradiation can reduce the risk of local recurrence [49]. This survival benefit is clearly observed in patients with lymph node positive and/or margin positive although an optimal adjuvant treatment strategy has not yet been established [32, 33]. The suggested treatment options by NCCN guidelines are fluoropyrimidine-based or gemcitabine-based chemotherapy or fluoropyrimidine chemoradiation followed by additional fluoropyrimidine or gemcitabine chemotherapy [33].

5. Advanced cholangiocarcinoma

Advanced distal cholangiocarcinoma, including locally advanced or metastatic, has overall poor prognosis. Most of them have obstructive jaundice due to biliary obstruction and they may also experience pruritus, pain, or cholangitis. Therefore, they are in need for palliative therapy to relieve their symptom, improve survival, and have a better quality of life.

Biliary drainage is indicated to relieve the symptom of biliary obstruction which will improve their quality of life and prepare some of those patients for chemotherapy. It can be obtained nonsurgically via endoscopic biliary drainage (EBD) or percutaneous transhepatic biliary drainage (PTBD). There is no difference between the two approaches in therapeutic success rate, overall complication, and 30 days mortality; however, PTBD has lower incidence of cholangitis [50, 51]. In regard to stent type, metallic stent is found to be better than plastic stent because it provides longer stent patency and lower risk of recurrent obstruction [52]. The classical way of biliary drainage is the surgical bypass with biliary-enteric anastomosis. Surgical bypass provides excellent relive of jaundice with low mortality and morbidity [53–55]. A meta-analysis of endoscopic versus surgical bypass in malignant biliary obstruction revealed no differences between surgical bypass and endoscopic plastic stents in the rates of technical success, therapeutic success, survival, and quality of life; however, the risk of all complication was in favor of plastic stent, and recurrent biliary obstruction was in favor of surgical bypass. But, the lower risk of biliary obstruction in surgical bypass is likely to result also in metallic stent. Therefore, nonsurgical stenting is the preferred first choice in malignant biliary obstruction in patients with short life expectancy. Surgical bypass can be considered in patients found to be unresectable during attempted curative resection and in patients with expected prolonged survival [4, 54, 56].

Systemic chemotherapy has proven to prolong the survival of advanced cholangiocarcinoma compared with best supportive care, with cisplatin/gemcitabine combination as a standard of care. Chemoradiation is another treatment strategy used for advanced cholangiocarcinoma, which provides effective local control and may prolong survival; however, it is recommended to patients with locally advanced disease without distant metastasis [33]. Photodynamic therapy is another local ablative technique that uses laser therapy to destruct bile duct cell cancer that has absorbed photosensitizing agent either through percutaneous transhepatic cholangiography or with ERC. It yields a good result in terms of increased survival benefit, improvement in biliary drainage, and better quality of life compared to biliary stent only [57, 58].

Author details

Ahmad Abdullah Madkhali* and Faisal Al-alem
Hepatobiliary Unit, Department of Surgery, College of Medicine, King Saud University, Riyadh, Saudi Arabia

*Address all correspondence to: ahmadmadkhali@gmail.com

References

[1] Vauthey JN, Blumgart LH. Recent advances in the management of cholangiocarcinomas. Seminars in Liver Disease. 1994;**14**(2):109-114

[2] DeOliveira ML, Cunningham SC, Cameron JL, et al. Cholangiocarcinoma: Thirty-one-year experience with 564 patients at a single institution. Annals of Surgery. 2007;**245**(5):755-762

[3] Lim JH. Cholangiocarcinoma: Morphologic classification according to growth pattern and imaging findings. American Journal of Roentgenology. 2003;**181**(3):819-827

[4] Moss AC, Morris E, Leyden J, MacMathuna P. Malignant distal biliary obstruction: A systematic review and meta-analysis of endoscopic and surgical bypass results. Cancer Treatment Reviews. 2007;**33**(2):213-221

[5] Kiriyama M, Ebata T, Aoba T, et al. Prognostic impact of lymph node metastasis in distal cholangiocarcinoma. The British Journal of Surgery. 2015;**102**(4):399-406

[6] Ito K, Ito H, Allen PJ, et al. Adequate lymph node assessment for extrahepatic bile duct adenocarcinoma. Annals of Surgery. 2010;**251**(4):675-681

[7] Hong SM, Pawlik TM, Cho H, et al. Depth of tumor invasion better predicts prognosis than the current American Joint Committee on cancer T classification for distal bile duct carcinoma. Surgery. 2009;**146**(2):250-257

[8] Zhou Y, Liu S, Wu L, Wan T. Survival after surgical resection of distal cholangiocarcinoma: A systematic review and meta-analysis of prognostic factors. Asian Journal of Surgery. 2017;**40**(2):129-138

[9] Chun YS, Pawlik TM, Vauthey JN. 8th Edition of the AJCC cancer staging manual: Pancreas and hepatobiliary cancers. Annals of Surgical Oncology. 2018;**25**(4):845-847

[10] Jun SY, Sung YN, Lee JH, Park KM, Lee YJ, Hong SM. Validation of the eighth American Joint Committee on cancer staging system for distal bile duct carcinoma. Cancer Research and Treatment. 2019;**51**(1):98-111

[11] Razumilava N, Gores GJ. Classification, diagnosis, and management of cholangiocarcinoma. Clinical Gastroenterology and Hepatology. 2013;**11**(1):13-21 e11. Quiz e13-14

[12] Chen CY, Shiesh SC, Tsao HC, Lin XZ. The assessment of biliary CA 125, CA 19-9 and CEA in diagnosing cholangiocarcinoma—The influence of sampling time and hepatolithiasis. Hepato-Gastroenterology. 2002;**49**(45):616-620

[13] Patel AH, Harnois DM, Klee GG, LaRusso NF, Gores GJ. The utility of CA 19-9 in the diagnoses of cholangiocarcinoma in patients without primary sclerosing cholangitis. The American Journal of Gastroenterology. 2000;**95**(1):204-207

[14] Choi JY, Kim MJ, Lee JM, et al. Hilar cholangiocarcinoma: Role of preoperative imaging with sonography, MDCT, MRI, and direct cholangiography. American Journal of Roentgenology. 2008;**191**(5):1448-1457

[15] Mansour JC, Aloia TA, Crane CH, Heimbach JK, Nagino M, Vauthey JN. Hilar cholangiocarcinoma: Expert consensus statement. The Official Journal of the International Hepato Pancreato Biliary Association. 2015;**17**(8):691-699

[16] Han JK, Choi BI, Kim AY, et al. Cholangiocarcinoma: Pictorial essay

of CT and cholangiographic findings. Radiographics. 2002;**22**(1):173-187

[17] Slattery JM, Sahani DV. What is the current state-of-the-art imaging for detection and staging of cholangiocarcinoma? The Oncologist. 2006;**11**(8):913-922

[18] Vilgrain V. Staging cholangiocarcinoma by imaging studies. The Official Journal of the International Hepato Pancreato Biliary Association. 2008;**10**(2):106-109

[19] Rizvi S, Gores GJ. Pathogenesis, diagnosis, and management of cholangiocarcinoma. Gastroenterology. 2013;**145**(6):1215-1229

[20] Hennedige TP, Neo WT, Venkatesh SK. Imaging of malignancies of the biliary tract—An update. Cancer Imaging. 2014;**14**:14

[21] Jhaveri KS, Hosseini-Nik H. MRI of cholangiocarcinoma. Journal of Magnetic Resonance Imaging. 2015;**42**(5):1165-1179

[22] Gulliver DJ, Baker ME, Cheng CA, Meyers WC, Pappas TN. Malignant biliary obstruction: Efficacy of thin-section dynamic CT in determining resectability. American Journal of Roentgenology. 1992;**159**(3):503-507

[23] Chung YE, Kim MJ, Park YN, et al. Varying appearances of cholangiocarcinoma: Radiologic-pathologic correlation. Radiographics. 2009;**29**(3):683-700

[24] Khan SA, Davidson BR, Goldin RD, et al. Guidelines for the diagnosis and treatment of cholangiocarcinoma: An update. Gut. 2012;**61**(12):1657-1669

[25] De Bellis M, Sherman S, Fogel EL, et al. Tissue sampling at ERCP in suspected malignant biliary strictures (part 1). Gastrointestinal Endoscopy. 2002;**56**(4):552-561

[26] Trikudanathan G, Navaneethan U, Njei B, Vargo JJ, Parsi MA. Diagnostic yield of bile duct brushings for cholangiocarcinoma in primary sclerosing cholangitis: A systematic review and meta-analysis. Gastrointestinal Endoscopy. 2014;**79**(5):783-789

[27] Blechacz B. Cholangiocarcinoma: Current knowledge and new developments. Gut and Liver. 2017;**11**(1):13-26

[28] Mohamadnejad M, DeWitt JM, Sherman S, et al. Role of EUS for preoperative evaluation of cholangiocarcinoma: A large single-center experience. Gastrointestinal Endoscopy. 2011;**73**(1):71-78

[29] Rerknimitr R, Angsuwatcharakon P, Ratanachu-ek T, et al. Asia-Pacific consensus recommendations for endoscopic and interventional management of hilar cholangiocarcinoma. Journal of Gastroenterology and Hepatology. 2013;**28**(4):593-607

[30] Garrow D, Miller S, Sinha D, et al. Endoscopic ultrasound: A meta-analysis of test performance in suspected biliary obstruction. Clinical Gastroenterology and Hepatology. 2007;**5**(5):616-623

[31] Sadeghi A, Mohamadnejad M, Islami F, et al. Diagnostic yield of EUS-guided FNA for malignant biliary stricture: A systematic review and meta-analysis. Gastrointestinal Endoscopy. 2016;**83**(2):290-298 e291

[32] Valle JW, Borbath I, Khan SA, et al. Biliary cancer: ESMO clinical practice guidelines for diagnosis, treatment and follow-up. Annals of Oncology. 2016;**27**(suppl 5):v28-v37

[33] Network NCC. Hepatobiliary Cancer (Version 1). 2019. Available from: https://www.nccn.org/professionals/physician_gls/pdf/hepatobiliary.pdf

[34] Fang Y, Gurusamy KS, Wang Q, et al. Meta-analysis of randomized clinical trials on safety and efficacy of biliary drainage before surgery for obstructive jaundice. The British Journal of Surgery. 2013;**100**(12):1589-1596

[35] Sewnath ME, Karsten TM, Prins MH, Rauws EJ, Obertop H, Gouma DJ. A meta-analysis on the efficacy of preoperative biliary drainage for tumors causing obstructive jaundice. Annals of Surgery. 2002;**236**(1):17-27

[36] Yao D, Kunam VK, Li X. A review of the clinical diagnosis and therapy of cholangiocarcinoma. The Journal of International Medical Research. 2014;**42**(1):3-16

[37] Komaya K, Ebata T, Shirai K, et al. Recurrence after resection with curative intent for distal cholangiocarcinoma. The British Journal of Surgery. 2017;**104**(4):426-433

[38] Jarnagin WR, Fong Y, RP DM, et al. Staging, resectability, and outcome in 225 patients with hilar cholangiocarcinoma. Annals of Surgery. 2001;**234**(4):507-517. Discussion 517-509

[39] Miyazaki M, Yoshitomi H, Miyakawa S, et al. Clinical practice guidelines for the management of biliary tract cancers 2015: The 2nd English edition. Journal of Hepato-Biliary-Pancreatic Sciences. 2015;**22**(4):249-273

[40] Chua TC, Saxena A. Extended pancreaticoduodenectomy with vascular resection for pancreatic cancer: A systematic review. Journal of Gastrointestinal Surgery. 2010;**14**(9):1442-1452

[41] Murakami Y, Uemura K, Hayashidani Y, et al. Prognostic significance of lymph node metastasis and surgical margin status for distal cholangiocarcinoma. Journal of Surgical Oncology. 2007;**95**(3):207-212

[42] Miyazaki M, Ohtsuka M, Miyakawa S, et al. Classification of biliary tract cancers established by the Japanese Society of hepato-biliary-pancreatic surgery: 3rd English edition. Journal of Hepato-Biliary-Pancreatic Sciences. 2015;**22**(3):181-196

[43] Ebata T, Yokoyama Y, Igami T, Sugawara G, Mizuno T, Nagino M. Review of hepatopancreatoduodenectomy for biliary cancer: An extended radical approach of Japanese origin. Journal of Hepato-Biliary-Pancreatic Sciences. 2014;**21**(8):550-555

[44] Zhou Y, Zhang Z, Wu L, Li B. A systematic review of the safety and efficacy of hepatopancreatoduodenectomy for biliary and gallbladder cancers. The Official Journal of the International Hepato Pancreato Biliary Association. Oxford: HPB; 2016 Jan;**18**(1):1-6. DOI: 10.1016/j.hpb.2015.07.008. [Epub 2015 Nov 30]

[45] Igami T, Nagino M, Oda K, et al. Clinicopathologic study of cholangiocarcinoma with superficial spread. Annals of Surgery. 2009;**249**(2):296-302

[46] Wakai T, Shirai Y, Moroda T, Yokoyama N, Hatakeyama K. Impact of ductal resection margin status on long-term survival in patients undergoing resection for extrahepatic cholangiocarcinoma. Cancer. 2005;**103**(6):1210-1216

[47] Ebata T, Yokoyama Y, Igami T, et al. Hepatopancreatoduodenectomy for cholangiocarcinoma: A single-center review of 85 consecutive patients. Annals of Surgery. 2012;**256**(2):297-305

[48] Xiang S, Lau WY, Chen XP. Hilar cholangiocarcinoma: Controversies on the extent of surgical resection aiming at cure. International Journal of Colorectal Disease. 2015;**30**(2):159-171

[49] Brandi G, Venturi M, Pantaleo MA, Ercolani G, GICO. Cholangiocarcinoma: Current opinion on clinical practice diagnostic and therapeutic algorithms: A review of the literature and a long-standing experience of a referral center. Digestive and Liver Disease. 2016;**48**(3):231-241

[50] Duan F, Cui L, Bai Y, Li X, Yan J, Liu X. Comparison of efficacy and complications of endoscopic and percutaneous biliary drainage in malignant obstructive jaundice: A systematic review and meta-analysis. Cancer Imaging. 2017;**17**(1):27

[51] Zhao XQ, Dong JH, Jiang K, Huang XQ, Zhang WZ. Comparison of percutaneous transhepatic biliary drainage and endoscopic biliary drainage in the management of malignant biliary tract obstruction: A meta-analysis. Digestive Endoscopy. 2015;**27**(1):137-145

[52] Yuan TW, Liu HQ, Wang SB, Cao J. Comparison of plastic stents with self-expandable metal stents in palliative treatment of malignant biliary obstruction: A meta-analysis. European Review for Medical and Pharmacological Sciences. 2017;**21**(12):2847-2857

[53] Kuhlmann KF, van Poll D, de Castro SM, et al. Initial and long-term outcome after palliative surgical drainage of 269 patients with malignant biliary obstruction. European Journal of Surgical Oncology. 2007;**33**(6):757-762

[54] Muller MW, Friess H, Koninger J, et al. Factors influencing survival after bypass procedures in patients with advanced pancreatic adenocarcinomas. American Journal of Surgery. 2008;**195**(2):221-228

[55] Nieveen van Dijkum EJ, Romijn MG, Terwee CB, et al. Laparoscopic staging and subsequent palliation in patients with peripancreatic carcinoma. Annals of Surgery. 2003;**237**(1):66-73

[56] Witzigmann H, Lang H, Lauer H. Guidelines for palliative surgery of cholangiocarcinoma. The Official Journal of the International Hepato Pancreato Biliary Association. 2008;**10**(3):154-160

[57] Leggett CL, Gorospe EC, Murad MH, Montori VM, Baron TH, Wang KK. Photodynamic therapy for unresectable cholangiocarcinoma: A comparative effectiveness systematic review and meta-analyses. Photodiagnosis and Photodynamic Therapy. 2012;**9**(3):189-195

[58] Lu Y, Liu L, Wu JC, Bie LK, Gong B. Efficacy and safety of photodynamic therapy for unresectable cholangiocarcinoma: A meta-analysis. Clinics and Research in Hepatology and Gastroenterology. 2015;**39**(6):718-724

Chapter 7

Surgical Treatment of Distal Common Bile Duct Malignancy

Adrian Bartos, Andrei Herdean and Dana Monica Bartos

Abstract

Distal cholangiocarcinoma is a rare malignant condition arising from the epithelial cells of the biliary tract. Surgical resection is the only curable alternative for patients with this disease. True resectability is often determined by surgical exploration. Duodenopancreatectomy is an extremely high-demanding technique and is the only one that can be potentially curable for patients diagnosed with resectable distal cholangiocarcinoma. Long-term survival may be achieved only in selected patients, undergoing duodenopancreatectomy, especially in patients where R0 margins are achieved. Perineural extension, pancreatic invasion, and lymph nodes involvement are the main risk factors for recurrence. Palliative biliodigestive diversion or endoscopic internal drainage of the biliary tree is alternative for patients with unresectable tumors. Although the prognosis after surgical treatment of distal common bile duct malignancy is better than for other periampullary tumors, the continuous progresses made in the field of surgical therapy and oncological treatment may lead to an improvement in the outcome of this neoplastic pathology.

Keywords: common bile duct tumors, surgical treatment, duodenopancreatectomy, jaundice palliation, laparoscopic pancreatic surgery

1. Introduction: general aspects

Biliary tract cancers are a group of neoplastic lesions originating from the epithelial cells of the biliary tract. This type of cancers are characterized by late diagnosis and also poor outcomes; they represent <1% of all cancers and approximately 3% of all gastrointestinal tumors [1] and affect elderly patients, especially men [2, 3]. Biliary tract cancers are categorized by their anatomical sites in distal, hilar, and intrahepatic cholangiocarcinoma. Intrahepatic cholangiocarcinoma is an entity defined by the fact that it is located proximally than the second-degree bile ducts. Perihilar cholangiocarcinoma represents the bile tract neoplasm characterized by the localization between the second-degree biliary ducts and the confluence between the cystic duct and the common bile duct. Distal cholangiocarcinoma is located from the confluence between the cystic duct and the common bile duct to the ampulla of Vater. Distal common bile duct cancer represents a periampullary neoplasm, which is less common than pancreatic adenocarcinoma, being very difficult to distinguish between them [2]. Most of the biliary tract neoplasms are adenocarcinomas, which can be well, moderately, and poorly differentiated. Other types are considered to be rare [4]. Five-year survival rate is extremely poor, despite the fact that surgery and liver transplantation represent options for selected candidates suffering from perihilar cholangiocarcinoma. Many patients are still not eligible for surgical treatment because of the advanced locoregional stage at the moment of diagnosis [1]. In order to obtain a higher survival rate, the multimodal treatment (surgery, chemotherapy, radiotherapy) should be considered in all stages of disease [5]. Regarding the chemotherapy, gemcitabine and cisplatin are usually used for treating inoperable cases. For intrahepatic cholangiocarcinoma, locoregional therapies were developed, but there is no conclusive evidence [2]. Perihilar localization is encountered in about 50% of the cases. The distal topography is found in approximately 40% of biliary tract cancers and the intrahepatic disease in less than 10% [6]. The epidemiology of these tumors is still poorly understood. Distal cholangiocarcinoma has a better prognosis and cure rate when compared to the pancreatic adenocarcinoma, but it still remains a high lethal medical condition. It is very important to make sure that a multidisciplinary approach is considered when dealing with distal cholangiocarcinoma [7].

2. Surgical treatment of distal cholangiocarcinoma: indications

2.1 Indications for radical treatment

Only a small number of patients are suitable for surgical treatment. In order to submit a patient for surgery, an assessment is mandatory, and it relies on accurate imaging and endoscopic techniques to assess the localization of the tumor and also the local and metastatic extent. In order to obtain an accurate staging and diagnosis, imaging should be done prior to biopsy. Ultrasound and CT are useful imaging tools for the staging of distal cholangiocarcinoma, but MRI with contrast angiography is the most accurate for assessing the biliary tract and the possible invasion of nearby vascular structures. The use of PET-CT scan is limited because of the presence of cholangitis, which can make the interpretation very difficult. The histological diagnosis is usually obtained by ERCP. The tissue sample can also be obtained by performing an endoscopic ultrasound with fine needle aspiration [8]. The selection of patients for surgery requires preoperative staging and surgical exploration (laparoscopy) in order to exclude the patients with unresectable or metastatic disease. A biopsy is not mandatory in the cases when there is a high index of suspicion [9].

In order to obtain the best long-term outcome, tumor resection with clear margins is mandatory. The main objective is represented by an aggressive resection strategy [10]. Distal cholangiocarcinomas encounter the highest rate of resectability when compared to hilar or intrahepatic cholangiocarcinomas [11]. The overall 5-year survival rate following curative surgery is between 16 and 52% in cases of distal cholangiocarcinoma. The operation generally requires a duodenopancreatectomy with typical reconstruction. In few cases, when the disease is extensively involving the biliary tract, a pancreaticoduodenectomy associated with a hepatic resection might be required. However, if there is a case of distant nodal extent, combined pancreatic and hepatic resections are not recommended due to the high morbidity and mortality rates that this operation presents. The guidelines recommend that a biliary drainage should be considered prior to radical resection in patients with jaundice. However, the need of biliary drainage should be assessed by a multidisciplinary team with high experience in dealing with distal cholangiocarcinomas [12].

2.2 Prognostic factors: operability criteria

There are two main predictors of survival after surgery: the status of surgical margins and lymph node involvement. Lymphadenectomy should be performed in the area of the pancreatic head and it is considered to be a vital part of the surgical intervention. Performing a frozen section examination of the proximal biliary tract margin should be considered in order to be sure that oncological surgical criteria are fulfilled [13, 14].

Resectability criteria:

- The absence of retropancreatic and paraceliac lymph nodal involvement
- The absence of liver metastases
- The absence of invasion of the main hepatic artery
- The absence of disseminated disease

3. Indications for palliative treatment: unresectable tumors

Locally advanced, unresectable, distal cholangiocarcinomas are divided into three main categories as it follows:

1. Microscopic positive margins (R1) after resection
2. Locally advanced, unresectable, from the moment of presentation
3. Recurrence after intent of curative treatment

The prognosis of unresectable cholangiocarcinomas is extremely poor: 6–12 months. The goal for these patients is to relieve symptoms and obtain a better quality of life. Also, it is well known that tumor debulking does not have a role and should be avoided in advanced cases of cholangiocarcinoma. Recently, chemotherapy combined with local therapies and biological therapies proved to be associated with a significant improvement in the survival rate. However, because of the rarity of the disease, many of these treatment options are assessed only in small studies and require to be validated by large prospective randomized trials [8]. Surgical treatment is contraindicated in cases of metastatic disease of the liver, lung, and peritoneum or in cases that present lymph nodes involvement beyond the head of the pancreas. Patients with unresectable or metastatic disease are considered for the palliation of jaundice. This is made either by a surgical bypass or, most frequently, by ERCP with the placement of a biliary stent. In cases of unresectable disease, a biopsy is mandatory in order to continue with any type of further treatment. Treatment options include the enrollment into a clinical trial, chemotherapy, radiotherapy, or chemoradiation procedures. There are trials that suggest the benefit of chemotherapy over best supportive care alone with reported overall survival rate of 9.5 versus 4.5 months [15, 16]. Another possibility for these patients is represented by chemoradiation. This way of treatment provides control of the symptoms and prolongs the overall survival rate. The most studied chemotherapeutic agent used in combination with radiotherapy was fluorouracil [17].

For patients with microscopically positive margins after surgery, the most recommended way of treatment consists of postoperative systemic chemotherapy combined with adjuvant chemoradiotherapy in conventional doses of radiation.

In cases of locally advanced and recurrent disease, the use of conventional doses of radiations has the role of relieving pain and may have a role in the decompression of the biliary tract [18].

Photodynamic therapy consists of intravenous injecting of a porphyrin photosensitizer combined with the endoscopic application of light on the tumor site.

This innovative technique leads to the death of the tumoral cell by generating free radicals of oxygen. Some studies suggest that photodynamic therapy combined with biliary decompression obtained after stenting provides a benefit in the overall survival rate of these patients [19–21]. Nowadays, photodynamic therapy is studied as a neoadjuvant condition. It is presumed that the rate of postoperative negative margins can be increased by submitting patients to neoadjuvant photodynamic therapy [22].

One of the most important aspects when dealing with locally advanced, unresectable, distal cholangiocarcinomas is represented by the palliation of jaundice. This can be realized by performing a surgical by-pass or by endoscopic placement of a stent. In patients who are found to suffer from an unresectable cholangiocarcinoma during a laparotomy, a surgical bypass is preferred. On the other way, in cases that the unresectable condition is diagnosed by imagining or laparoscopy, the endoscopic placement of a biliary stent is preferred. In most cases, the palliation of jaundice is obtained by an endoscopic approach [23, 24]. The most common relapse pattern is represented by local recurrence. Positive margins and lymph node involvement are predictive risk factors for local recurrence. The typically sites of metastases are the liver and the peritoneum.

4. Surgical technique and approach

4.1 Duodenopancreatectomy

Duodenopancreatectomy represents a very complex surgical intervention. It is performed in cases of resectable periampulary tumors: distal cholangiocarcinoma, tumors of the pancreatic head, tumors of the ampulla of Vater, and tumors of the duodenum [25].

The surgical intervention begins with either a median or bilateral subcostal incision (in thin patients, a median incision is preferred). First important step during a duodenopancreatectomy is to search for distant metastases. Once the surgeon rules out the presence of liver or peritoneal metastases, the Kocher maneuver is performed in order to identify the relation of the tumor with the retroperitoneal structures and especially the superior mesenteric artery. The superior mesenteric artery is dissected beginning from the right side of the Treitz's ligament, in order to exclude the tumoral involvement of the artery. This procedure is known as artery-first approach. Access to the omental bursa is gained by the division of the gastrocolic ligament. In order to mobilize the hepatic flexure of the colon, careful dissection of the avascular plane located between the hepatic flexure and the duodenum must be performed. Once the colonic flexure is mobilized caudally, the Kocher maneuver can be extended in order to allow the access to the D3 portion of the duodenum (**Figure 1**). Now, the gastroepiploic vein is divided and the superior mesenteric vein appears on the inferior margin of the pancreas. In order to complete this step of the surgical intervention, a tunnel is made between the neck of the pancreas and the portal vein (**Figure 2**). Further, the dissection continues in the supraduodenal region as it follows. Cholecystectomy is performed in the classical way. After the dissection of the Callot triangle, the common bile duct is divided just proximal from the origin of the cystic duct. After the cystic artery is identified, it is closed by ligation and divided. A very important step for obtaining best oncological outcome is represented by the lymphadenectomy of the hepatoduodenal ligament continued toward the celiac trunk. During this dissection, the proper hepatic artery, originating from the common hepatic artery and the main branches of the celiac trunk, can be isolated. The gastroduodenal artery is now divided near its origin (**Figure 3**). In order to obtain the preservation of the pylorus (optional step), the right

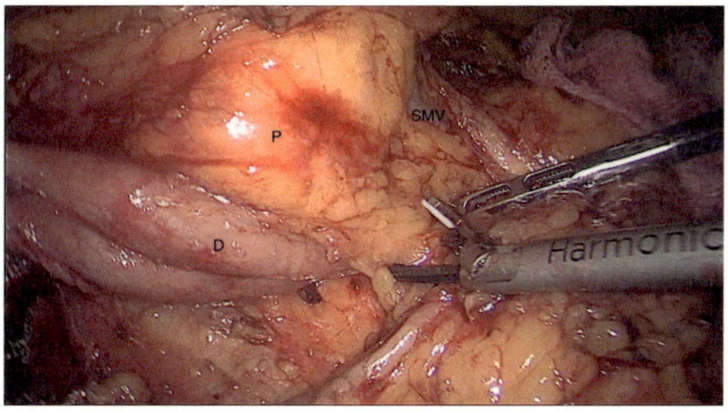

Figure 1.
Kocher maneuver; laparoscopic approach (from the personal archive of the authors). P = pancreatic head; D = duodenum; SMV = superior mesenteric vein.

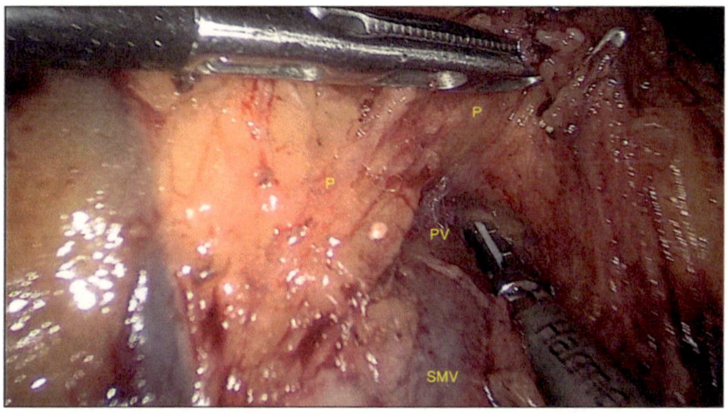

Figure 2.
Dissection of the SMV and PV from the pancreatic isthmus; laparoscopic approach (from the personal archive of the authors). P = pancreatic head; SMV = superior mesenteric vein; PV = portal vein.

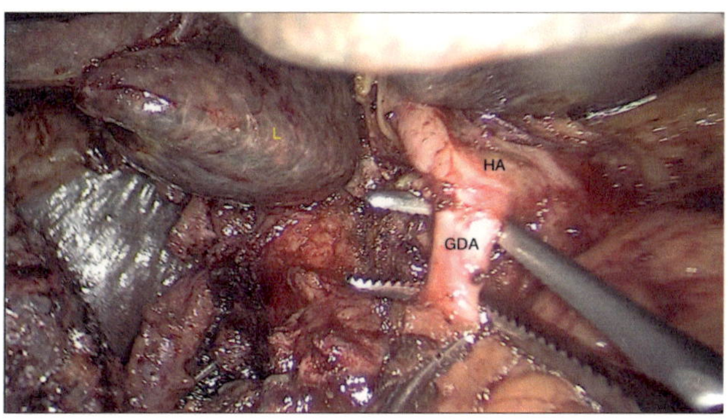

Figure 3.
Dissection of the gastroduodenal artery; laparoscopic approach (from the personal archive of the authors). L = liver; HA = hepatic artery; GDA = gastroduodenal artery.

gastric and right gastroepiploic arteries should be divided. After the mobilization of the first 2 cm of the duodenum is performed, the portal vein is widely exposed. The superior and inferior pancreatic vessels are now ligated by placing two sutures on both the superior and inferior borders of the pancreas. Those two sutures are extremely important for minimizing the bleeding after transection of the pancreas. A tunnel is now fully created between the portomesenteric trunk and the posterior surface of the pancreatic neck. The Treitz angle and the first jejunal loop are now

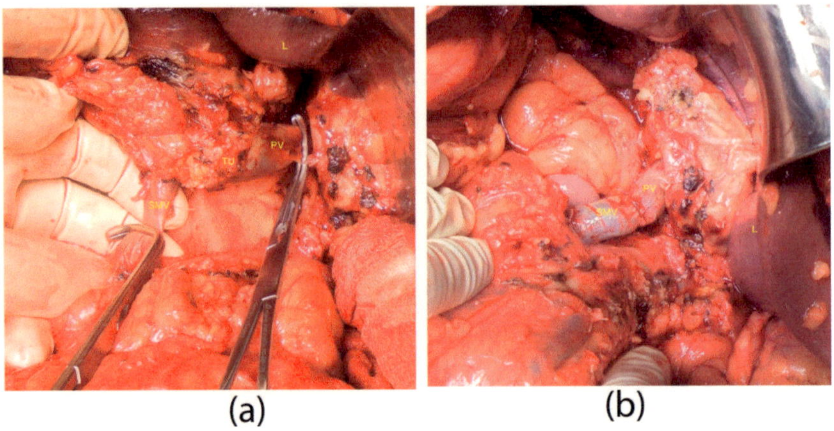

Figure 4.
Vascular resection of a tumor with invasion in the portal vein; open approach (from the personal archive of the authors). L = liver; PV = portal vein; SMV = superior mesenteric vein; TU = tumor. (A) Before vascular resection; and (B) after vascular reconstruction.

dissected and divided so that the jejunum can be tractioned into the supramesocolic compartment. The dissection along the superior mesenteric artery and vein is carefully performed using a bipolar electrocautery and clips or ligatures. The venous (portal, superior mesenteric, venous confluent) resection, if required, is performed in the last step (**Figure 4A** and **B**). By gently retracting the portal vein, in order to expose the retroportal tissue, the venous branches that drain directly into the portal vein are identified, ligated, and divided. The transection of the pancreatic neck is now performed by using a scalpel (classic or harmonic). It is very important to obtain a perfect hemostasis at the level of the pancreatic stump. This is obtained by placing nonabsorbable monofilament sutures. Some authors consider that by using the bipolar or monopolar cautery, an insecure hemostasis is obtained and also the pancreatic tissue can be damaged, the fact that may compromise future anastomosis. As a final step of the extirpative phase, the duodenum (in pylorus preserving technique) is divided using a linear stapler. Now the specimen is removed and sent for histopathological examination. The pancreatic stump is now mobilized in order to obtain a tension-free pancreatic anastomosis (with the stomach or the jejunum). The second main phase of this very complex operation is the reconstructive phase. Now, in order to obtain the continuity of the digestive tract, three anastomoses must be performed. Firstly, the pancreatic stump is anastomosed either with the stomach (posterior surface) or the jejunum. As long as the basic principle of a safe anastomosis is considered, any technique may be successful. The bilioenteric anastomosis is performed usually as an end to side single layer anastomosis (**Figure 5**). Another important aspect is that the bilioenteric anastomosis is performed on the antimesenteric margin of the jejunum. The final reconstruction is represented by the gastrojejunostomy (or duodenojejunostomy if pylorus preserving technique was used). Most authors prefer an antecolic gastrojejunostomy performed at approximately 50 cm downstream from the biliodigestive anastomosis.

Finally, abdominal drains and nasogastric tube are placed. A feeding jejunostomy may now be performed. After a final evaluation of hemostasis, the musculoaponeurotic plane is closed and the skin is sutured.

4.2 Palliative surgery

There are different surgical approaches in order to obtain jaundice palliation. However, these procedures are rarely performed due to the fact that they were largely replaced by endoscopic placing of stents [26].

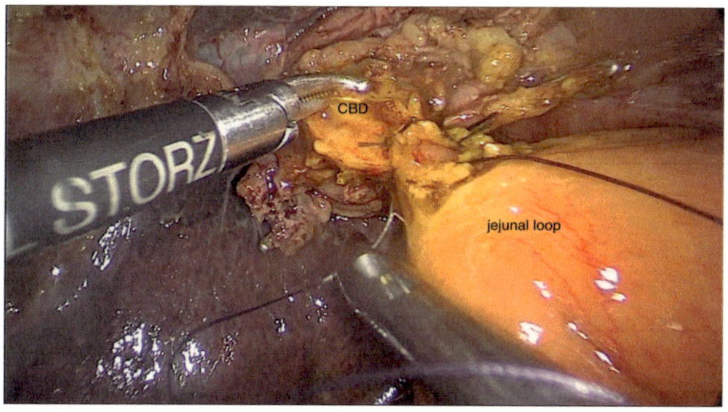

Figure 5.
Biliojejunal anastomosis; laparoscopic approach (from the personal archive of the authors). CBD = common bile duct.

In order to perform a bilioenteric bypass, the *cholecystectomy* is a mandatory step. The most important moment in performing the cholecystectomy is the dissection of Callot triangle, where the elements of the gallbladder pedicle are located. The isolation, ligation, and resection of the cystic duct and artery are performed at this level. The next step of the procedure is the dissection of the gallbladder from its hepatic fossa using the electrocautery or scissors.

4.2.1 Choledochoduodenostomy

Choledochoduodenostomy is a useful operative technique when dealing with unresectable distal cholangiocarcinoma. After performing a cholecystectomy, a supraduodenal longitudinal choledochotomy is performed and the biliary tract is explored. By performing a wide Kocher maneuver, the duodenum can be mobilized in order to obtain a tension-free anastomosis. A longitudinal duodenotomy is performed on the D1 portion of the duodenum. Two corner sutures are placed between the ends of the duodenotomy and the middle parts of the choledochotomy. Another corner suture is placed between the inferior pole of the choledochotomy and the midposterior point of the duodenotomy. Now the posterior raw of sutures is applied and tied. Next, the forth corner suture is applied between the superior pole of the choledochotomy and the midanterior point of the duodenotomy. This makes it easier to perform the anterior layer of sutures. Like other biliodigestive anastomosis, single-layer sutures are recommended (**Figure 6**) [26].

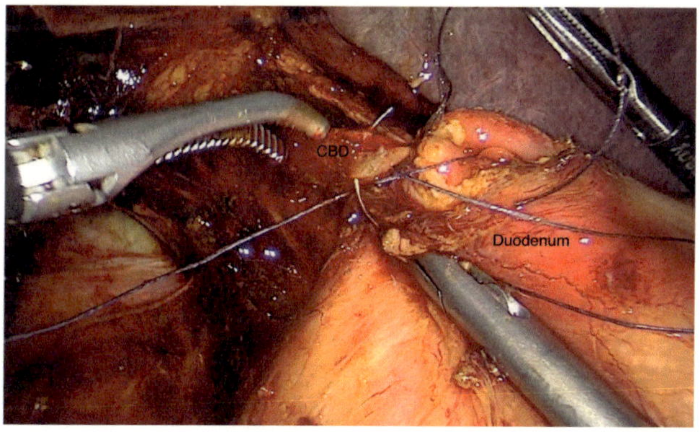

Figure 6.
Side-to-side choledochoduodenostomy for unresectable neoplasia; laparoscopic approach (from the personal archive of the authors). CBD = common bile duct.

4.2.2 Choledochojejunostomy and hepaticojejunostomy

A hepaticojejunostomy can be performed either on the left or the right hepatic ducts. This surgical intervention is performed through a right subcostal incision. Extending the incision toward the xiphoid process or with a left subcostal incision provides a good approach in order to perform the biliary-enteric bypass. By removing the gallbladder, a better access to the extrahepatic biliary ducts is gained.

In order to approach the left hepatic duct, the teres ligament is divided to obtain a better exposure of the left hemiliver. On the visceral surface of the left hemiliver, the left hepatic duct goes together with the left branch of the portal vein and they are found together into a peritoneal reflection. The best way to gain access in this area is by lowering the hilar plate.

On the other hand, the right hepatic duct can be approached by dissecting along the base of IVb segment of the liver. In this way, the biliary confluent is well visualized. As it often happens, the right hepatic duct is too short in length and small hepatic parenchyma incisions may be needed in order to visualize the intrahepatic right portal pedicle.

Once the access is gained, a 60–70 cm Roux en Y jejunal loop is prepared and delivered through a breach in the mesocolon located on the right from the middle colic pedicle. The posterior row of sutures is now performed in order to secure the duct mucosa to the jejunal mucosa. With the anterior sutures retracted upward, the posterior row is now tied up. Further, the anterior row is completed by suturing the jejunal mucosa. Finally, the anterior layer is tied and the anastomosis is complete [26].

In order to perform a choledochojejunostomy, the technique is the same, except the location on the common bile duct where the anastomosis is done.

4.2.3 Endoscopic and percutaneous drainage

If the malignant disease is too advanced and a surgical curative treatment is not suitable, biliary drainage needs to be established in order to lower the effects of hyperbilirubinemia. Percutaneous transhepatic drainage and endoscopic retrograde cholangiopancreatography are widely used for the palliation of jaundice.

Percutaneous transhepatic biliary drainage is a procedure performed under fluoroscopic or ultrasound guidance. With increased expertise and better instrumentation, the technical success rate is of ~90–95% with fewer complications rates [27].

ERCP is accepted as the preferred procedure worldwide as it is a comparably safer procedure with relatively fewer contraindications. Absolute contraindications for ERCP are as follows: pharyngeal or esophageal obstruction and active coagulopathy [28, 29]. This procedure also has some relative contraindications, such as the presence of acute pancreatitis or severe cardiopulmonary disorder. Unlike percutaneous transhepatic drainage, burden of percutaneous drainage catheter and bag is obviated, which further compounds the psychological burden of terminally ill patients. In the current scenario, in cases of distal common bile duct obstruction, ERCP is the preferred technique unless contraindicated, for which the percutaneous approach is performed [27].

5. Results

Despite the fact that biliary tract cancer is associated with a high mortality rate, patients diagnosed with distal cholangiocarcinoma have a better survival rate when compared with other periampullary cancers. The poor prognosis is due to the fact that many patients are suffering from an advanced stage at the time of surgery; this is proved by the high incidence of lymph node involvement, perineural extension, and lymphatic and vascular invasion [30]. Significant improvement of short-term outcome has been encountered lately due to the development of surgical techniques and perioperative management. Nowadays, it is considered that the mortality rate following surgery is less than 5%, when talking about high-volume centers [30, 31]. The 5-year overall survival rate is now considered to range from 13 to 54%. The poor prognosis is due to the fact that biliary tract cancer encounters two main forms of extension: submucosal spreading and superficial spreading. Those two cause the high rate of positive margins obtained in surgery. This is why an intraoperative frozen examination of the margins is extremely important [30]. If R0 resection is performed, the overall survival rate at 5 years is considerably increased from 0–40% (R1 margins) to 27–60% (R0 margins) [30, 32]. Surgeons worldwide make efforts to improve the prognosis of this disease. Some of them claim that extended lymphadenectomy combined with the dissection of nerve plexus surrounding major blood vessels improves the outcome [30]. However, there are still a lot of controversies around this strategy. A very controversial aspect is represented by postoperative adjuvant chemotherapy. There are studies that show no significant difference in the 5-year overall survival rate between those who receive adjuvant chemotherapy (gemcitabine, paclitaxel, oxaliplatin, fluorouracil) when compared to those who have not [33]. In order to establish significant prognostic factors for distal cholangiocarcinoma, several studies were conducted. They assessed prognostic factors such as perineural extent, lymph node involvement, and the histological differentiation of the tumor. Studies that analyze the prognostic factors for 5-year overall survival rate of patients diagnosed with distal cholangiocarcinoma and submitted to surgery with curative intent conclude that the presence of R1 margins, lymph node involvement, perineural invasion, lymphatic and vascular extension, pancreatic invasion, and the presence of tumors >T3 is associated with poor prognosis. Those studies conclude that obtaining R0 margins substantially improves the outcome and is one of the most important prognostic factors [30]. In order to obtain better outcome, more accurate diagnostic modalities should be developed.

6. Future perspectives

Laparoscopic duodenopancreatectomy represents one of the most advanced abdominal interventions and it still has small widespread so far (**Figures 1–3, 5, 7**). The complexity of this procedure is due to the facts that dissection of the portal vein, lymphadenectomy, and dissection of the uncinate process are extremely high demanding. When comparing to other minimally invasive procedure, the rate of conversion is higher. This is due to the adhesions to large vascular structures and uncontrollable bleeding. Reported rates of conversion are ranging between 0 and 40%. The difference between the reported rates of conversion arises from the liberalization of intraoperative decision to convert [34]. The mean operating time is significantly longer during minimally invasive duodenopancreatectomies when compared to the open procedure. In addition to the complexity of the resection step, performing the reconstructive step is technically high demanding and of course, time-consuming. It is considered that the learning curve extends for several years, in order to obtain good outcome [35, 36]. Hybrid approach might be a solution in order to accumulate experience. In this type of surgical approach, the anastomoses are performed through a small laparotomy [33, 34]. Hybrid approach is considered to provide a safely development to a totally laparoscopic method [37]. The learning curve can be shortened by practicing simple sutures and then gastrointestinal anastomoses on the simulator or animal models. There are studies that

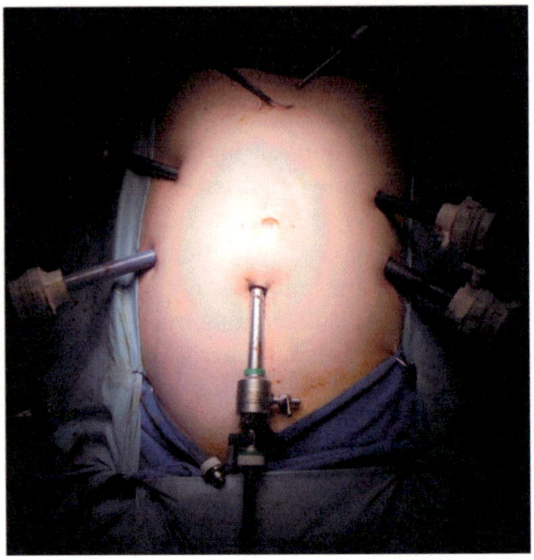

Figure 7.
Port placement for laparoscopic duodenopancreatectomy (from the personal archive of the authors).

demonstrate favorite outcomes in case of using a robotic and laparoscopic hybrid approach. In this case, the resection is performed laparoscopically and then, with robotic assistance, the surgeon performs the reconstructive step [38]. Data showed a lower blood loss in the minimally invasive approach when compared to the open technique. As a consequence, there is a lower need of transfusion, which is an objective outcome. However, there is a high risk of perioperative morbidity and mortality, the fact that limits the development of minimally invasive duodenopancreatomy. Literature concludes that the open approach has a morbidity rate between 23 and 66% with a mortality of 3–5% in high-volume centers [39, 40]. The minimally invasive technique has a morbidity ranged between 18.2 and 87.5% with a mortality rate of 0–6.9%, comparable to the open approach. The main complication following duodenopancreatectomies is considered to be pancreatic fistula. There are comparable rates of complications (severe pancreatic fistula, delayed gastric emptying, pancreatic stump hemorrhage) when comparing the open technique with minimally invasive [41], the fact that encourages to consider the use of the minimally invasive approach as safe as the open technique. However, it is necessary that large prospective studies to be done, in order to obtain a comparison between these two techniques regarding long-term outcomes such as survival rate and quality of life [42].

The use of robotics may turn useful in promoting the application of a minimally invasive approach in major procedures in the treatment of distal cholangiocarcinoma. Robotic surgery has proven to be feasible, but its oncologic adequacy is yet to be demonstrated by larger studies.

7. Key points

- Jaundice is the most important clinical manifestation of this neoplastic disease.
- Surgical resection is the only curable alternative for patients with distal cholangiocarcinoma.
- The treatment of choice for resectable tumors is duodenopancreatectomy.

- Duodenopancreatectomy can be performed either open or laparoscopically, in high-volume centers.
- The palliation of jaundice is the cornerstone for treatment of the advanced distal cholangiocarcinoma.
- Long-term survival may be achieved only in selected patients, undergoing duodenopancreatomy, especially in patients where R0 margins are achieved.
- Perineural extension, pancreatic invasion, and lymph nodes involvement are the main risk factors for recurrence.

Acknowledgements

Adrian Bartoş is the coordinator of this chapter.

Author details

Adrian Bartos[1]*, Andrei Herdean[1] and Dana Monica Bartos[1,2]

1 Surgical Department, "Prof. Dr. Octavian Fodor" Regional Institute of Gastroenterology and Hepatology, Cluj-Napoca, Romania

2 Anatomy Department, "Iuliu Hatieganu" University of Medicine, Cluj-Napoca, Romania

*Address all correspondence to: bartos.adi@gmail.com

References

[1] Waseem D, Tushar P. Intrahepatic, perihilar and distal cholangiocarcinoma: Management and outcomes. Annals of Hepatology. 2017;**16**(1):133-139

[2] Razumilava N, Gores GJ. Cholangiocarcinoma. Lancet. 2014;**383**(9935):2168-2179

[3] Squadroni M, Tondulli L, Gatta G, Mosconi S, Beretta G, Labianca R. Cholangiocarcinoma. Critical Reviews in Oncology/Hematology. 2017;**116**:11-31

[4] Blechacz B, Gores GJ. Cholangiocarcinoma: Advances in pathogenesis, diagnosis, and treatment. Hepatology. 2008;**48**(1):308-321

[5] Bonet Beltran M, Allal AS, Gich I, Sole JM, Carrio I. Is adjuvant radiotherapy needed after curative resection of extrahepatic biliary tract cancers? A systematic review with a meta-analysis of observational studies. Cancer Treatment Reviews. 2012;**38**(2):111-119

[6] DeOliveira ML, Cunningham SC, Cameron JL, Kamangar F, Winter JM, Lillemoe KD, et al. Cholangiocarcinoma: Thirty-one-year experience with 564 patients at a single institution. Annals of Surgery. 2007;**245**(5):755-762

[7] Dickson PV, Behrman SW. Distal cholangiocarcinoma. Surgical Clinics of North America. 2014;**94**(2):325-342

[8] Skipworth JR, Keane MG, Pereira SP. Update on the management of cholangiocarcinoma. Digestive Diseases. 2014;**32**(5):570-578

[9] Cho A, Yamamoto H, Kainuma O, Muto Y, Yanagibashi H, Tonooka T, et al. Laparoscopy in the management of hilar cholangiocarcinoma. World Journal of Gastroenterology. 2014;**20**(41):15153-15157

[10] Endo I, Gonen M, Yopp AC, Dalal KM, Zhou Q, Klimstra D, et al. Intrahepatic cholangiocarcinoma: Rising frequency, improved survival, and determinants of outcome after resection. Annals of Surgery. 2008;**248**(1):84-96

[11] Miura F, Sano K, Amano H, Toyota N, Wada K, Yoshida M, et al. Evaluation of portal vein invasion of distal cholangiocarcinoma as borderline resectability. Journal of Hepato-Biliary-Pancreatic Sciences. 2015;**22**(4):294-300

[12] Ribero D, Zimmitti G, Aloia TA, Shindoh J, Fabio F, Amisano M, et al. Preoperative cholangitis and future liver remnant volume determine the risk of liver failure in patients undergoing resection for Hilar cholangiocarcinoma. Journal of the American College of Surgeons. 2016;**223**(1):87-97

[13] Qiao QL, Zhang TP, Guo JC, Zhan HX, Zhao JX, Liu YC, et al. Prognostic factors after pancreatoduodenectomy for distal bile duct cancer. The American Surgeon. 2011;**77**(11):1445-1448

[14] Ito K, Ito H, Allen PJ, Gonen M, Klimstra D, D'Angelica MI, et al. Adequate lymph node assessment for extrahepatic bile duct adenocarcinoma. Annals of Surgery. 2010;**251**(4):675-681

[15] Sharma A, Dwary AD, Mohanti BK, Deo SV, Pal S, Sreenivas V, et al. Best supportive care compared with chemotherapy for unresectable gall bladder cancer: A randomized controlled study. Journal of Clinical Oncology: Official Journal of the American Society of Clinical Oncology. 2010;**28**(30):4581-4586

[16] Geynisman DM, Catenacci DV. Toward personalized treatment of advanced biliary tract cancers. Discovery Medicine. 2012;**14**(74):41-57

[17] Czito BG, Anscher MS, Willett CG. Radiation therapy in the treatment of cholangiocarcinoma. Oncology. 2006;**20**(8):873-884. Discussion 86-8, 93-5

[18] Sahai P, Kumar S. External radiotherapy and brachytherapy in the management of extrahepatic and intrahepatic cholangiocarcinoma: Available evidence. The British Journal of Radiology. 2017;**90**(1076):20170061

[19] Moole H, Tathireddy H, Dharmapuri S, Moole V, Boddireddy R, Yedama P, et al. Success of photodynamic therapy in palliating patients with nonresectable cholangiocarcinoma: A systematic review and meta-analysis. World Journal of Gastroenterology. 2017;**23**(7):1278-1288

[20] Lu Y, Liu L, Wu JC, Bie LK, Gong B. Efficacy and safety of photodynamic therapy for unresectable cholangiocarcinoma: A meta-analysis. Clinics and Research in Hepatology and Gastroenterology. 2015;**39**(6):718-724

[21] Fuks D, Bartoli E, Delcenserie R, Yzet T, Celice P, Sabbagh C, et al. Biliary drainage, photodynamic therapy and chemotherapy for unresectable cholangiocarcinoma with jaundice. Journal of Gastroenterology and Hepatology. 2009;**24**(11):1745-1752

[22] Wagner A, Wiedmann M, Tannapfel A, Mayr C, Kiesslich T, Wolkersdorfer GW, et al. Neoadjuvant down-sizing of Hilar cholangiocarcinoma with photodynamic therapy-long-term outcome of a phase II pilot study. International Journal of Molecular Sciences. 2015;**16**(11):26619-26628

[23] Heedman PA, Astradsson E, Blomquist K, Sjodahl R. Palliation of malignant biliary obstruction: Adverse events are common after percutaneous transhepatic biliary drainage. Scandinavian Journal of Surgery: Official Organ for the Finnish Surgical Society and the Scandinavian Surgical Society. 2018;**107**(1):48-53

[24] Shariff MI, Khan SA, Westaby D. The palliation of cholangiocarcinoma. Current Opinion in Supportive and Palliative Care. 2013;**7**(2):168-174

[25] Werner J, Büchler MW. Chapter 62A: Resectional techniques: Pancreaticoduodenectomy, distal pancreatectomy, segmental pancreatectomy, total pancreatectomy, and transduodenal resection of the papilla of Vater. In: Jarnagin WR, Blumgart LH, editors. Blumgart's Surgery of the Liver, Pancreas and Biliary Tract. 5th ed. Philadelphia: W.B. Saunders; 2012. pp. 945-966.e3

[26] Cho CS, MI D'A. Chapter 29: Bile duct exploration and biliary-enteric anastomosis. In: Jarnagin WR, Blumgart LH, editors. Blumgart's Surgery of the Liver, Pancreas and Biliary Tract. 5th ed. Philadelphia: W.B. Saunders; 2012. pp. 470-480.e1

[27] Chandrashekhara SH, Gamanagatti S, Singh A, Bhatnagar S. Current status of percutaneous transhepatic biliary drainage in palliation of malignant obstructive jaundice: A review. Indian Journal of Palliative Care. 2016;**22**(4):378-387

[28] Mohammad Alizadeh AH. Cholangitis: Diagnosis, treatment and prognosis. Journal of Clinical and Translational Hepatology. 2017;**5**(4):404-413

[29] Silviera ML, Seamon MJ, Porshinsky B, Prosciak MP, Doraiswamy VA, Wang CF, et al. Complications related to endoscopic retrograde cholangiopancreatography: A comprehensive clinical review. Journal of Gastrointestinal and Liver Diseases. 2009;**18**(1):73-82

[30] Zhou Y, Liu S, Wu L, Wan T. Survival after surgical resection of distal

cholangiocarcinoma: A systematic review and meta-analysis of prognostic factors. Asian Journal of Surgery. 2017;**40**(2):129-138

[31] Hong SM, Pawlik TM, Cho H, Aggarwal B, Goggins M, Hruban RH, et al. Depth of tumor invasion better predicts prognosis than the current American Joint Committee on Cancer T classification for distal bile duct carcinoma. Surgery. 2009;**146**(2):250-257

[32] Kwon HJ, Kim SG, Chun JM, Lee WK, Hwang YJ. Prognostic factors in patients with middle and distal bile duct cancers. World Journal of Gastroenterology. 2014;**20**(21):6658-6665

[33] Wellner UF, Shen Y, Keck T, Jin W, Xu Z. The survival outcome and prognostic factors for distal cholangiocarcinoma following surgical resection: A meta-analysis for the 5-year survival. Surgery Today. 2017;**47**(3):271-279

[34] Wang Y, Bergman S, Piedimonte S, Vanounou T. Bridging the gap between open and minimally invasive pancreaticoduodenectomy: The hybrid approach. Canadian Journal of Surgery. 2014;**57**(4):263-270

[35] Shyr B-U, Chen S-C, Shyr Y-M, Wang S-E. Learning curves for robotic pancreatic surgery-from distal pancreatectomy to pancreaticoduodenectomy. Medicine. 2018;**97**:45

[36] Rodríguez-Sanjuán JC, Gómez-Ruiz M, Trugeda-Carrera S, Manuel-Palazuelos C, López-Useros A, Gómez-Fleitas M. Laparoscopic and robot-assisted laparoscopic digestive surgery: Present and future directions. World Journal of Gastroenterology. 2016;**22**(6):1975-2004

[37] Zureikat AH, Breaux JA, Steel JL, Hughes SJ. Can laparoscopic pancreaticoduodenectomy be safely implemented? Journal of Gastrointestinal Surgery: Official Journal of the Society for Surgery of the Alimentary Tract. 2011;**15**(7):1151-1157

[38] Ji W, Ding K, Kao X, He C, Li N, Li J. Robotic and laparoscopic hybrid pancreaticoduodenectomy: Surgical techniques and early outcomes. Chinese Medical Journal. 2014;**127**(16):3027-3029

[39] Elberm H, Ravikumar R, Sabin C, Abu Hilal M, Al-Hilli A, Aroori S, et al. Outcome after pancreaticoduodenectomy for T3 adenocarcinoma: A multivariable analysis from the UK Vascular Resection for Pancreatic Cancer Study Group. European Journal of Surgical Oncology. 2015;**41**(11):1500-1507

[40] de Wilde RF, Besselink MG, van der Tweel I, de Hingh IH, van Eijck CH, Dejong CH, et al. Impact of nationwide centralization of pancreaticoduodenectomy on hospital mortality. British Journal of Surgery. 2012;**99**(3):404-410

[41] Xiong JJ, Tan CL, Szatmary P, Huang W, Ke NW, Hu WM, et al. Meta-analysis of pancreaticogastrostomy versus pancreaticojejunostomy after pancreaticoduodenectomy. British Journal of Surgery. 2014;**101**(10):1196-1208

[42] Chen K, Pan Y, Liu X-L, Jiang G-Y, Wu D, Maher H, et al. Minimally invasive pancreaticoduodenectomy for periampullary disease: A comprehensive review of literature and meta-analysis of outcomes compared with open surgery. BMC Gastroenterology. 2017;**17**(1):120